Also by Ted and Larry:

- <u>Simple as ABG</u> – so healthcare students could finally understand <u>A</u>rterial <u>B</u>lood <u>G</u>ases.
- And, coming soon, <u>R U Still Medically Curious?</u> about heart attacks, strokes, media myths, and all those supplement claims.

SECOND EDITION

R U MEDICALLY CURIOUS?

Simple Answers to Common Medical Questions

Dr. Larry Romane

EDITED BY TED HEYMAN

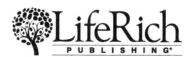
LifeRich
PUBLISHING

LifeRich Publishing is a registered trademark of The Reader's Digest Association, Inc.

LifeRich Publishing books may be ordered through booksellers or by contacting:

LifeRich Publishing
1663 Liberty Drive
Bloomington, IN 47403
www.liferichpublishing.com
1 (888) 238-8637

Because of the dynamic nature of the Internet, any web addresses or links contained in this book may have changed since publication and may no longer be valid. The views expressed in this work are solely those of the author and do not necessarily reflect the views of the publisher, and the publisher hereby disclaims any responsibility for them.

Any people depicted in stock imagery provided by Thinkstock are models, and such images are being used for illustrative purposes only. Certain stock imagery © Thinkstock.

Any people depicted in stock imagery provided by Shutterstock are models, and such images are being used for illustrative purposes only. Certain stock imagery © Shutterstock.

ISBN: 978-1-4897-0716-1 (sc)
ISBN: 978-1-4897-0717-8 (e)

Library of Congress Control Number: 2016904795

Print information available on the last page.

LifeRich Publishing rev. date: 04/07/2016

*Special thanks to David Ray Fink for his
great help with photography.

TOPICS

INTRODUCTION

<u>R U MEDICALLY CURIOUS?</u> Not just a little, but **really** curious? You spend your whole life in the same body. Yet, most of you know almost nothing about it. As a physician, what always intrigued me were my patients' **questions**. Otherwise very bright people seemed absolutely clueless in medical matters. It's not for lack of information. The Media and the Internet supply tons of that – both good and bad. No, the problems are language and understanding.

Here's how it works: I take your history, do a physical exam, and review your tests. Then, I slowly nod my head as I tell you my diagnosis. To be polite, you slowly nod your head, even when you have no idea what I just said. Your mothers would be proud. You always nod politely.

So, **language** is the first problem and doctors get full blame. We created a whole new secret lingo called "Medicalese". It's not your thigh bone. It's your *Femur*. You didn't have a heart attack. You had an *Acute Myocardial Infarction*. Even a simple toothache might be an *Anaerobic Gingival Abscess!* (see Chapter 3 – Translating Medicalese)

But, not **understanding?** You get full credit for that one. Why? The Media and Internet feed you a steady diet of medical oddities, rarities, and misleading information. You swallow those like vintage champagne. You eagerly discuss them with all your friends. But, when's the last time you pushed your doctor so you could understand something? Hmmm… Old saying: An expert who can't explain his expertise is not an expert.

R U MEDICALLY CURIOUS? is written at a high school reading level to present Evidence Based Medicine on common medical topics.

TED is Ted Heyman, the Editor. He's a computer guy from Florida who's known Larry since high school. He edited Larry's respiratory textbook Simple as ABG and created the e-version of it.

LARRY is me, Dr. Larry Romane. I'm board certified in Emergency Medicine, worked as an ER doc for 35 years, retired, and now teach and write about medicine.

Can **you** answer these simple medical questions in 10 words or less?

- What's a 'Carpal Tunnel'? Does it charge a toll?
- What's 'Medicalese' and why can't I speak it?
- Aren't brand name medicines safer than generics?
- Why is everybody I know getting Diabetes?
- My diet is terrible. Shouldn't I be on some vitamin or supplement or something?

If not, maybe you're more medically curious than you thought.

APOLOGY: Sorry healthcare professionals, this book is **not** for you. It's written for laymen. You'll say "it's over-simplified", "numbers are rounded off", "pictures are only schematics", "averages can be misleading", etc. And... you're RIGHT! (But, before you get too condescending, please review the "References" section at the back of the book.)

WEIGHT TIPS, Q-TIPS, MORE TIPS

OK, medical stuff can be pretty complicated. Let's leave Diabetes, Orthopedics, Medications, etc. for later. But, since <u>Webster's</u> defines a tip as a "helpful hint", let's start with 'Health Tips'.

WEIGHT TIPS

One third of all Americans are obese. Another one third are overweight. (See Height/ Weight chart at end of this chapter) When 2/3's of the population weighs too much, it begins to look 'normal'. Things like Diabetes, High Blood Pressure, and knee replacements should remind us - it's definitely **not** normal.

Q: Who wrote the most definitive medical article on weight loss in the last 20+ years? (OK – in my opinion)

A: In 2009, Harvard's Dr. Frank Sacks published his diet research in the "New England Journal of Medicine". The title was "Comparison of Weight Loss Diets with Different Compositions of Fat, Protein, and Carbohydrate" [1] (for details, see OUR DIABETIC EPIDEMIC). Conclusion: It's not **what** you eat but how many **calories** you eat. Period! Even the *FDA* (**F**ood & **D**rug **A**dministration) finally agrees. For the first time in 20 years they're changing that "Nutrition Facts" label on all packaged foods. "Calories" and "Serving Size" are now more prominent.

Nutrition Facts

Serving Size 1 cup (110g)
Servings Per Container About 6

Amount Per Serving

Calories 250	Calories from Fat 30

	% Daily Value*
Total Fat 7g	**11%**
Saturated Fat 3g	**16%**
Trans Fat 0g	
Cholesterol 4mg	**2%**
Sodium 300mg	**13%**
Total Carbohydrate 30g	**10%**
Dietary Fiber 3g	**14%**
Sugars 2g	
Protein 5g	

Vitamin A	7%
Vitamin C	15%
Calcium	20%
Iron	32%

* Percent Daily Values are based on a 2,000 calorie diet. Your daily value may be higher or lower depending on your calorie needs.

	Calories:	2,000	2,500
Total Fat	Less than	55g	75g
Saturated Fat	Less than	10g	12g
Cholesterol	Less than	1,500mg	1,700mg
Total Carbohydrate		250mg	300mg
Dietary Fiber		22mg	31mg

Nutrition Facts

6 servings per container

Serving Size   1 cup (110g)

Amount per 1 cup

Calories   250

% DV*	
11%	**Total Fat** 7g
16%	**Saturated Fat** 3g
	Trans Fat 0g
2%	**Cholesterol** 4mg
13%	**Sodium** 300mg
10%	**Total Carbs** 30g
14%	**Dietary Fiber** 3g
	Sugars 2g
	Added Sugars 0g
	Protein 5g

7%	**Vitamin A** 1mcg
15%	**Vitamin C** 2mcg
20%	**Calcium** 4mg
32%	**Iron** 5mg

* Percent Daily Values are based on a 2,000 calorie diet. Your daily value may be higher or lower depending on your calorie needs.

	Calories:	2,000	2,500
Total Fat	Less than	55g	75g
Saturated Fat	Less than	10g	12g
Cholesterol	Less than	1,500mg	1,700mg
Total Carbohydrate		250mg	300mg
Dietary Fiber		22mg	31mg

A few weight loss tips:

- A pound of fat contains about 3,500 calories. Cutting back 100 calories every day for a year, takes off about 10 pounds.
- 3 basic food groups: carbohydrates, proteins, and fats. Carbohydrates and proteins have the **same** calories per ounce. An ounce of dietary fat has **double** the calories.
- Exercise is great for your heart, your blood pressure, your brain, etc. But, the human body is a very efficient machine. Exercise only burns about 200-300 calories per hour.
- 2 body parts cause 98+% of overweight and obesity. The *Thyroid Gland* and the hands. If a simple *TSH* Thyroid test is normal, you're hands are putting too many calories in your mouth.

METRIC TIPS

Yes, The American Metric Association was founded in 1916. Yes, President Gerald Ford signed "The Metric Conversion Act" into law in 1975. Yes, the American Metric Association renamed itself the "U.S. Metric Association". Yes, its 300 members are still working to convert us.[2] And, yes, the metric system is a sound, scientific way to describe lengths, weights, and volumes.

Sorry guys, after almost a century of your best efforts, mainstream America will not budge. But, just enough Metric remnants remain to drive us crazy. Here are some approximate conversions if you ever need them:

VOLUME:

2 Tablespoons = 30 cc's (cubic centimeters) = 1 ounce

LENGTH: Inches (in.) and Centimeters (cm.) 1 inch = 2.5 centimeters

EXAMPLE: 4 inches = ? centimeters. Multiply 4 inches by 2.5 = 10 cm. So, 4 in. = 10 cm

WEIGHT: To change Pounds (lbs.) to Kilograms (Kg.) Divide Pounds in half, then subtract 10%

EXAMPLE: 100 lbs. = ? Kg. Divide 100 lbs. in half = 50

10% of 50 = 5

Subtract 5 from 50 = 45

So, 100 lbs. = 45 Kg

(Remember, I said "approximate conversions". With a calculator, 100 lbs. is really **45**.454545…Kg. But, my 45 Kg conversion is still more accurate than your bathroom scale.)

———————

————

RADIATION

Background: Diagnostic x-rays come in 2 basic types:

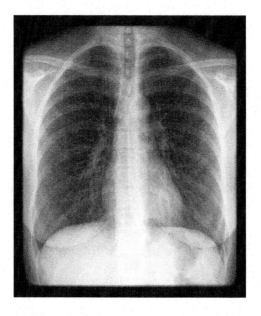

Plain Film: X-ray beam goes thru a body part from front to back or side to side. Like Superman looking through you. Good News? Less radiation. Bad News? Less detail for the radiologist to read.

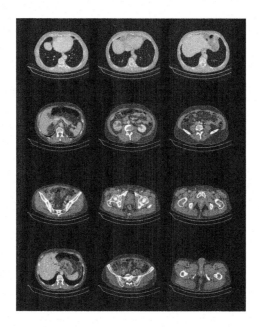

CAT Scan (CT Scan for short): X-ray beam slices the body crosswise like a meat slicer in a deli. Good News? Shows more tissues in more detail. Bad news? **Much** more radiation.

Like most things, too much of anything is not good. That's true with radiation. X-rays may disrupt the genetic information in the nucleus of a cell. That can kill the cell – like Radiation Therapy for cancer. Even a little too much radiation may cause future DNA changes in a cell – leading to cancer decades in the future.

Two things determine radiation injury - quantity and patient age. Quantity is easy – the greater the radiation, the greater the danger. Patient age is also simple. If cancer from radiation doesn't show up for decades, be worried about x-raying 2 year olds, not 80 year olds.

Rads, Roentgens, and Sieverts are all scientific scales to measure radiation. Forget them! Everyone's had at least one chest x-ray in their life. Let's use that for our scale – the amount of radiation in one chest x-ray:

CAT Scan of Head – about 100 Chest X-rays worth of radiation

CAT Scan of Chest – about 200 Chest X-rays

CAT Scan of Abdomen and Pelvis – about 500 Chest X-rays

Dental X-ray – 1/20th the radiation of a Chest X-ray

Airport Screening X-ray – 1/1000th of a Chest X-ray

MRI means **M**agnetic **R**esonance **I**maging and contains **no** x-ray radiation.

Crystal Ball: the very newest CAT scanners will have "ultra-low" radiation. Good News? Better than Plain Films for diagnosis **and** less radiation. Bad News? $$$ to replace all inexpensive plain x-rays with more expensive CAT scans!

BITE WOUNDS

We own about 70 million dogs and 75 million cats.[3] We also get more than 5 million mammal bites every year[4] costing over $100 million for treatment! What bites are most likely to get infected? About 5% of dog bites get infected, 60% of cat bites, and 90+% of **human** bites. Another reason why dogs are man's best friend.

Rabies - Bad News first: In human history, probably only 8 survivors of active rabies infection. Good News? 100 years ago, rabies killed about 100 Americans per year. That number is now 2-3 deaths per year. Why the drop?

- In the 1940's we started vaccinating dogs against rabies. Cat vaccines came later. Those shots eliminated a huge reservoir for potential rabies. Today, the highest wild animal bite risks are skunks, foxes, bats, and raccoons.

RABIES 'BIG 4'

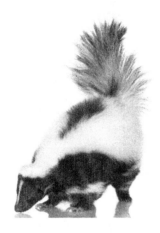

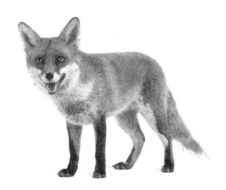

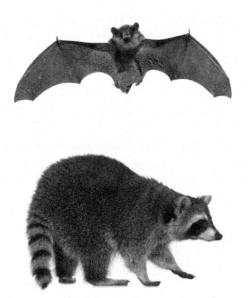

- Don't worry about bites from rodents or rabbits. They can **get** rabies but they don't **transmit** the disease.
- We now have both active and passive anti-rabies injections for patients at risk.[5] You get 1 passive immunity shot immediately and 3 active immunity shots over the next year. They're so good you'll still have 97% immunity in 10 years.[6]

CHILD-PROOF MEDICINE BOTTLES

As a retired ER doctor, I know safety lids make young children safer. As a senior citizen, I know they're a pain in the butt! Arthritic fingers weren't meant for "Press down and turn". Need help?

1. Place bottle near edge of table.

2. Grasp bottle firmly with right hand.
3. Press left palm down on bottle cap.
4. Keep left elbow against waist.
5. Lean body weight down on left hand.
6. Rotate your whole body to the left.
7. *Voila!*

Or, no young kids around your home? Just ask your pharmacist for 'Snap On Lids'.

———————
————

ALCOHOL – NECTAR OF THE GODS?

Alcohol has been around since ancient times. Drunken chariot drivers were killing people long before there were drunken motorists.

Wine? Whiskey? Beer? Regardless of what form it's in, we like the feeling. In fact, a little may even be beneficial. Most risk assessments for heart attack or stroke list "1-2 drinks per day" as a positive influence.

Ah, there's the rub. Exactly what is 'a drink'? It's **not,** "just a 6 pack, doc". **Nor** is it, "just a little Jack on ice, Your Honor". 'A Drink' is:

- **One** 12 oz. can of beer or
- **One** shot of 80 proof whiskey (1 ½ oz.) or
- **One** 5 oz. glass of wine.

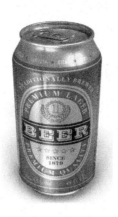

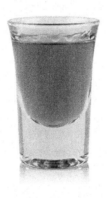

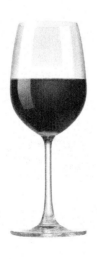

About the same alcohol in all three!

What about alcohol and driving? Remember, my specialty is Emergency Medicine. I know what drunk drivers do. I liked the idea of ignition keys tied to car breathalyzers.

- Q: Can a 175 lb. man legally drive after 4 beers watching a Sunday NFL game? **NO.**
- Q: Can a 135 lb. woman legally drive after 3 glasses of wine at a 2 hr. lunch? **NO.**
- Don't believe it? Try this website: **bloodalcoholcalculator.org**. Enter your weight, sex, number of beers or drinks, and time you've been drinking. You'll get a good guestimate of your blood alcohol level.

Here's how Maryland does it: When you get pulled over, you get a field sobriety test. Next comes a breathalyzer to determine your blood alcohol. This is where it gets confusing. Sane people know they shouldn't drive drunk. Drunk drivers don't know this because they're… DRUNK.

DUI used to mean Driving Under the Influence. **DWI** meant Driving While Intoxicated. Individual state laws now make those terms a problem. Here's what you need to know: If you blow a 0.04 – 0.07, you **are** an impaired driver. Forget your explanations and be as polite as possible. Your driver's license, your money, and/or your liberty are about to take a hit. If, on the other hand, your breathalyser is 0.08 or higher, you're **drunk**. Shut up, cooperate while they put on your handcuffs, and try not to stagger or fall down. Forget your money and your license - you're too late. Concentrate on how to spend as little time locked up as possible.

Suppose your DUI or DWI caused an accident? Here's the kind of guy who drives drunk and hurts people. Do you really think taking away that little plastic driver's license will stop him? When we catch an armed robber, we don't give him back his pistol. Why does the drunk driver get his car back? You're shocked. Suppose it was a $250,000 Ferrari? At auction, that should really help lower my taxes.

BAD BODY SMELLS

Yuck. Nice topic, right? Bad breath and body odor are unique medical conditions. They're the only ones that bother bystanders more than they bother the patient.

Halitosis is the medical term for bad breath. Sure, it can be from something you ate (garlic), something you drank (alcohol), or something you inhaled (tobacco smoke). You already know those. One Question: Is offending others enough to make you change things you like? Your choice. Halitosis is **not** from those things and usually comes from mouth infections. An infected tooth is easy. It's usually sensitive to cold or actually hurts. Plan: See your dentist. More commonly, bad breath comes from bacteria under inflamed gums - *Gingivitis*.

Background: bacteria come in 2 types – aerobic bacteria love oxygen while **an**aerobic bacteria hate oxygen **and** really stink. Just give an anaerobe a warm, moist, dark place with poor circulation (low oxygen) and he's happy. Throw in some rotting leftover food morsels stuck under the gums and he's in heaven.

Plan: Try a new toothbrush. Sound wave toothbrushes (sonic or ultrasonic) move their bristles **30,000** times a minute[7] - or more! Try to match that with your hand toothbrush. Compared to hand brushing, they can be **twice** as effective at reducing inflamed gums and gum bleeding. They're also **5** times more effective at removing dental *plaque*.[8] That's the sticky film of dissolved foods and mouth bacteria that covers your teeth. If it isn't removed, it hardens into *tartar* paving the way for both tooth and gum disease.

B.O. is slang for Body Odor. If there's an official medical term, I can't find it. Again, you need some background. We have two different kinds of sweat glands: *Apocrine* and *Epocrine.*

Apocrine sweat is just salt water secreted by your skin when you overheat. Lick your fingertip. Now blow on it. Fingertip got cooler, right? Evaporation causes cooling. That's why you sweat. Apocrine sweat usually has no odor (unless you ate something like lots of garlic).

Epocrine sweat is different. It has waxy fats mixed with the salt water. Remember those anaerobic bacteria in your mouth? How they love warm, dark, moist places? How they're always smelly? The bacteria turn the fats rancid. Hair follicles in your armpit and crotch are made to order for these guys.

Plan: Shower daily with **any** anti-bacterial soap. And, be sure your underarm product is both antiperspirant **and** deodorant.

Oh, one last bad smell. Your kid's got a snotty nose – but only on **one** side. It really stinks. He or she probably stuck something up the nostril. Guess what? It's probably still there.

———————

————

CLEANING EARS WITH Q-TIPS

3 good reasons to **never** 'clean' your ears with Q-Tips:

- Ear wax is as normal in your ear canals as saliva is on your lips – and just as protective. The wax is secreted by cells deep in the canal, dirt and dust stick to it, daily cell growth pushes the wax out the canal, showering washes it away when it gets to the outside. Perfect design.
- Shoving a Q-Tip down a tapering funnel makes no sense. You push **in** more wax than you get **out**. You may even push it right thru your eardrum (bad idea)

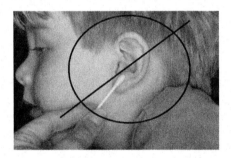

- *Otitis externa* – 'Swimmer's Ear' is a painful, smelly, draining infection of the ear canal. What starts it? First, Q-tips wipe away protective wax. Then, they scratch and scrape the delicate canal lining. Finally, water from the 'ole swimmin' hole may not be exactly sterile… As the "International Journal of Pediatric Otolaryngology" put it, "Use of cotton tip applicators to clean the ear seems to be the leading cause of otitis externa in children and should be avoided."[9]

Side Note: this is one of the few **bacterial** infections that usually doesn't need an antibiotic. Most doctors prescribe ear drops that combine a dilute vinegar solution (acetic acid) and hydrocortisone. Bacteria can't stand the new acidity in the canal. Meanwhile, hydrocortisone helps the pain and inflammation.

DRIVERS USING CELL PHONES

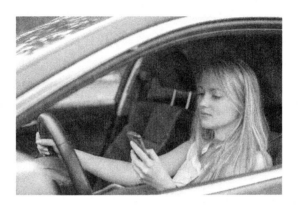

Yes, I'm sure this doesn't apply to **you**. You're a perfect driver, but...

1. For years, we've known that using a cell phone while driving increases your risk of an *MVA* (**M**otor **V**ehicle **A**ccident). That increased risk is about **4 times as great**.
2. Drivers under 20 have better eyes and faster reflexes. Yet their risk of an MVA driving using a cell phone is reported at **6 fold.** (Why? Driving inexperience, overconfidence, frequency of cell phone use, texting, etc.)
3. If you initiate the call while driving, the risk begins 2+ minutes **before** you call (thinking about the call, finding the phone, entering a number while going through the red light, etc.)
4. And **NO**, hands-free phones do **not** improve your risk.
5. **5 seconds** – average time a driver's eyes are off the road while texting. At 60 mph, you cover **1 ½ football fields** in that time. Texting while driving is about the same risk as drunk driving. (References for 1-5 = [10,11,12,13])

QUESTION: Why don't we prosecute texting drivers like we do drunk drivers?

———————

————

DEHYDRATION

Oxygen is our #1 essential nutrient. Without it, you start to die in 5-6 minutes.

What's our #2 nutrient? Yes….this section is called "Dehydration". You got it. **Water's** our #2 essential nutrient. Without water, death occurs in less than a week. Add the heat and dryness of a desert? You may not make it 24 hours without water. The more free water you had in your body to start with, the longer you can last.

But, not everyone has the same amount of body water. The average adult's weight is about 2/3's water. So, a 150 lb. man has about 100 lbs. of water. This varies widely. Newborn infants may be 75% water. Obese bodies may only have 48% – 50% water by weight.[14]

It's said that every human biochemical reaction requires at **least** 1 water molecule. Dehydration simply means you don't have enough water. Symptoms parallel how low your water supply has gotten:

- You're 5% dry or less: When your Extra Cellular Fluid (mostly water) drops 5% you'll have decreased skin *Turgor*. What's that? Skin has lots of fluid. Pinch your forehead. When you let go, the fluid content immediately eliminates the pinch mark. If you're dehydrated, the skin stays pinched a few seconds.

- 5-10% dehydrated: When you stand, your pulse speeds up and your blood pressure drops. Why? Your body is asking you to lie down and your heart is pumping your remaining fluid around as fast as it can.
- Dehydration over 10%: There's not enough fluid to pump around the oxygen and nutrients you need. Symptoms? Very fast heart rate. Very low blood pressure. Rapid breathing. Confusion. Medical term for this? *SHOCK*[15]

Causes?

- Hot environment – body loses water in sweat to try to cool down.
- Exercise – same water loss.
- Stomach problems like vomiting and diarrhea - prevent water intake and retention.
- Medications – first line blood pressure medications often cause fluid loss, as do other drugs.

Treatment?

Oral fluids if you can take them, IV fluids if you can't. What fluids? Sweat is **not** water. It's dilute **salt** water. No wonder NFL players grab for Gatorade and athletes fondly call it "lime flavored sweat". Remember, fluids with caffeine or alcohol **don't** count. They're diuretics and can make you pee out more than you just drank.

Whole House Dehydration: It's Winter. Chapped lips, dry hands, clogged nose, scratchy throat, and static electricity. Ever wonder why? In Winter, the heat's on in a sealed house. "The relative humidity in the Sahara Desert is 25% and the average home is 13-15%".[16] Treatment requires 2 purchases: Inexpensive humidifier for at least your bedroom and cheap Hygrometer to measure humidity. Aim for 40% relative humidity, that's comfortable. Higher levels mean mold and mildew could be your new roommates.

MELANOMA's A, B, C, & D

MELANOMA: A very dangerous skin cancer. Early treatment has over 95% cure rate. Late disease is almost always fatal. Most common in fair-skinned patients with a family history of melanoma[21]. As with most skin cancers, sun exposure is a key risk. Any suspicious or changing lesion needs biopsy.

Melanoma's 4 Classic Warning Signs are A, B, C, and D[22]:

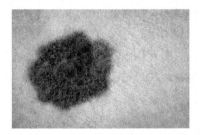

'A' stands for Asymmetry: Lesion can't be divided into 2 equal halves.*

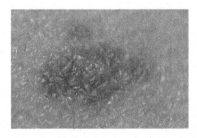

'B' stands for Border: Border is irregular, not round.*

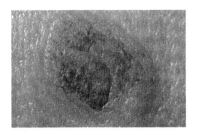

'C' stands for Color: Lesion has several colors.*

*See great color images at shutterstock.com

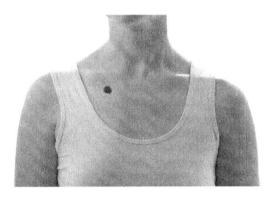

'D' stands for Diameter: Bigger than a pencil eraser (6mm).

GLOBAL WARMING

Wait, I need my helmet before you read this one. 1.9 million years ago our poor planet had its first Ice Age. Since then, there have been at least 4 more. Each time, Earth warmed up enough to melt the ice and move on. So really, Global Warming isn't new. The last melt was about 25,000 years ago[17]. Man was around, but not in numbers or development to make much difference. Now, scientific experts and research data tell us Earth is warming up again. The reason seems to be rising amounts of "Greenhouse Gases". Among those, Carbon Dioxide (CO_2) and Water Vapor (H_2O) seem to be top culprits. These, in turn, come from burning fossil fuels. Fossil fuels are hydrocarbons, abbreviated CHO. That means they contain Carbon (C), Hydrogen (H), and Oxygen (O). When hydrocarbons are ignited in the presence of Oxygen, you get Energy and 2 'exhaust' products – carbon dioxide and water vapor. The equation for that is pretty easy:

$$\textbf{CHO (fossil fuel) + O}_2 \textbf{ = ENERGY + CO}_2 \textbf{ + H}_2\textbf{O}$$

With me so far? OK, all fossil fuels are hydrocarbons (CHO's). But, all hydrocarbons are **not** fossil fuels. What hydrocarbons **aren't** fossil fuels? Just about everything we eat - meats, seafood, fruits, nuts, dairy products, etc. Yes, they're all very different chemicals. But, they're all Carbon-Hydrogen-Oxygen based. We eat them as 'fuel' to run our engine. What's the equation for that?

$$\textbf{CHO (food) + O}_2 \textbf{ = ENERGY + CO}_2 \textbf{ + H}_2\textbf{0}$$

Hmmm….anybody notice that burning fossil fuel and burning the food we eat are the exact same equation? Let's start with that CO_2 we exhale as exhaust. Normal CO_2 in Earth's atmosphere is about 0.04%.[18] Human exhaled air has 4.0% CO_2.[19] That's a **100 fold** increase every time you breathe out. Each of us exhales about 720 **pounds** of CO_2 per year. Before you say, "Wow, that's scary.", remember 3 things about humans:

- Before we exhale, we saturate inhaled air with water vapor (as in Greenhouse Gas #2)
- Before we exhale, we raise inhaled air temperature to about 98.6 F (remember, our topic is Global **Warming**)
- Finally, remember *homo sapiens* passed a milestone in 2013 – there are now 7 **billion** of us exhaling 12-15 times every minute.

"The fault, dear Brutus, is not in our stars, but in ourselves…"[20]

National Weight Guidelines *

Height (feet, inches)	Overweight (pounds)	Obese (pounds)
5' 0"	128	153
5' 1"	132	158
5' 2"	136	164
5' 3"	141	169
5' 4"	145	174
5' 5"	150	180
5' 6"	155	186
5' 7"	159	191
5' 8"	164	197
5' 9"	169	203
5' 10"	174	209
5' 11"	179	215
6' 0"	184	221
6' 1"	189	227

Normal Weight = Body Mass Index (BMI) 19 - 25
Overweight = Body Mass Index (BMI) 25 - 30
Obese = Body Mass Index (BMI) 30 and over

*This chart is compiled from data on the National
Institutes of Health's "Body Mass Index Table 1".
(www.nhlbi.nih.gov/health/educational)

OUR DIABETIC EPIDEMIC:
SUGAR, SUGAR EVERYWHERE

Definition: Diabetes is too high blood sugar from too little insulin.

The medical term is *Diabetes Mellitus* (mellitus is honey in Latin). So, doctors often abbreviate Diabetes as DM. If the patient requires insulin, the abbreviation is IDDM. That stands for **I**nsulin **D**ependent **D**iabetes **M**ellitus.

Just how big is the problem? America has 317 million people. 26 million of us already have Diabetes.[1] Another 79 million are estimated to have *Pre-Diabetes*.[2] That means they're on a ledge and just about to fall off. That's a potential for one third of all Americans to become diabetic.

Next, let's take that word sugar. Blood sugar is **not** table sugar. Table sugar is *Sucrose*. Blood sugar is *Glucose*. Confused?

OK. All sugars are carbohydrates. And, sugars come in 2 types – Simple and Complex.

SIMPLE SUGARS are basic carbohydrate building blocks, like Legos. Examples:

1. *Glucose* – It's our #1 energy source, our fuel. It's ready for use anytime, anywhere - if you have enough insulin. (see below)
2. *Fructose* - That's the simple sugar found in almost all fruits. It's sweeter than glucose.

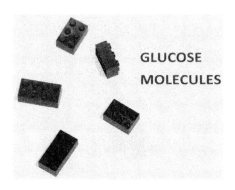

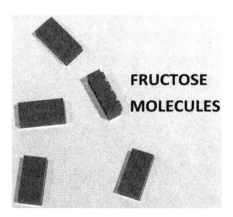

COMPLEX SUGARS are just simple sugars hooked together. Examples:

1. *Sucrose* – That's table sugar. It's 50% glucose + 50% fructose. (*High Fructose Corn Syrup* is similar but has 5% more fructose).
2. *Honey* – Another complex sugar made of - you guessed it – **Fructose** and **Glucose.** Honey's 38% fructose and 31% glucose. What's the remainder? About 17% water, 13% other sugars, and 0.5% minerals, enzymes, vitamins, etc.[3] Question: If fructose is so terrible, why hasn't anybody notified the bees?

(Contrary to media hype, **neither** fructose **nor** sucrose contribute to obesity or increased appetite any more than any other nutrient with the same calories[4,5,6])

3. *Glycogen* – Here's a really complex sugar. It's **30,000** glucose molecules linked together. The liver makes glycogen for long term energy storage.

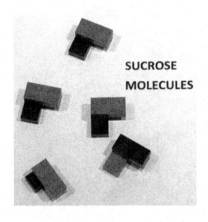

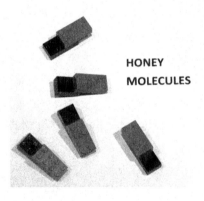

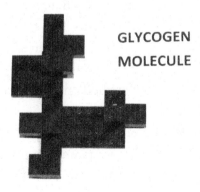

Now, back to Diabetes. Since blood sugar is glucose, then diabetics have too much glucose in their blood. So what? Statistics are boring, but:

Each year, 230,000 Americans die with "Diabetes" written on their death certificate (that's over **5 times** as many as breast cancer)[7,8]

- Diabetes **triples** your risk for heart attack and stroke.
- Diabetes is the leading cause of kidney failure (Imagine dialysis 3 times a week for life).
- Diabetes is the leading cause of **blindness** after age 20.
- Diabetic healthcare costs 2 ½ times that of non-diabetics.[9] Think our economy can handle that?

————————

————

Remember the definition of Diabetes. Diabetes is **high** blood sugar (glucose) from too little insulin. What's a **normal** sugar? (Measured either fasting or at least 2 hours after eating)

- Normal glucose is 70-99.
- Pre-Diabetes is a glucose of 100-125.
- Diabetes is defined as blood glucose over 125.[10]

Your question should be, "Well, what causes Diabetes?" Someday researchers or geneticists may be able to tell us. So far, all we know is that Diabetes comes in 2 Types. Each type has different **theories** about its cause.

Before we get to Type I and Type II, you need a little background. Diabetes is NOT a sugar disease. It's an insulin disease. What's insulin? Insulin is a hormone made in the pancreas to regulate blood sugar. The pancreas is an *Endocrine* (hormone) organ located in the belly, behind the stomach.

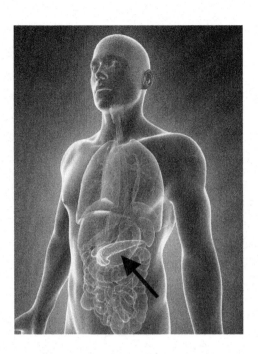

Compare your body to an automobile. For a car, crude oil is refined to gasoline; gasoline is pumped into the engine; the engine mixes gasoline with oxygen; a spark plug ignites the mixture; ENERGY is created.

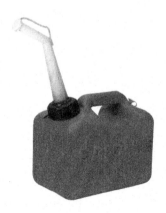

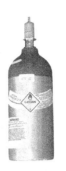

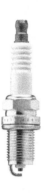

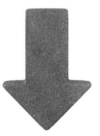

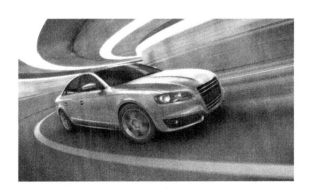

In humans, our daily food is refined (digested) to glucose; insulin moves the glucose into our cells and "burns" it with oxygen; ENERGY is created.

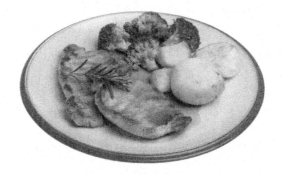

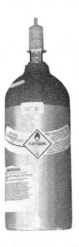

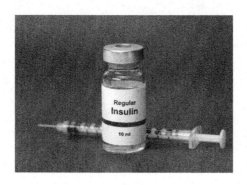

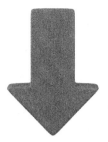

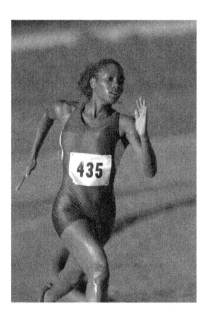

Now, back to those two **Types** of Diabetes. Currently, *Type I Diabetes* and *Type II Diabetes* are the best terms to use. Names like Juvenile and Adult Onset Diabetes are no longer correct (see why, below). Here's the breakdown:

Type I Diabetics have NO insulin. These patients are usually children or young adults. One day, an otherwise healthy person suddenly starts destroying the *Beta Cells* in his own pancreas. Beta cells make insulin. The current theory for this is called ***Auto-immune Disorder***.

The immune system that usually protects us goes awry. It now sees the pancreas' beta cells as foreign invaders and destroys them. No beta cells = no insulin. Without insulin, blood sugar rises rapidly. A normal glucose of 100 soars to several hundred or even 1000. That triggers a complex chemical nightmare and severe symptoms. (see SYMPTOMS, below).

Glucose can't be burned for energy because there's no insulin. In desperation, the body tries burning fat instead. In our overweight society, burning fat sounds good, right? Not exactly.

When we burn glucose, our 'exhaust' is carbon dioxide - CO_2. Just exhale and you're fine. But, fat is an 'alternate fuel' that doesn't burn clean. The exhaust from burning fat is *Acetone*. That's right, acetone, as in nail polish remover – a very serious poison.

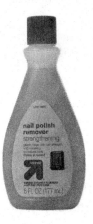

In severe cases, you can even smell acetone on the patient's breath. He needs immediate IV fluids and insulin. Without that treatment, he'll die in the first 24 - 48 hours. Afterward, he'll be an IDDM (Insulin Dependent Diabetic) for life. A pancreas transplant someday is his only hope.

GOOD NEWS? Type I Diabetes had been declining for over 15 years. No idea why…Unfortunately, new cases of both Type 1 and Type 2 are now **increasing** in children.

Type II Diabetics seem to have a normal pancreas making normal insulin. They just can't make **enough** insulin for their needs. Two theories try to explain why:

Insulin Resistance Theory: This one is currently in vogue. For some reason, cells suddenly need more insulin than they used to. They've become resistant to insulin's effects. 2 big problems: 5 national diabetic organizations can't agree on a definition or cause for insulin resistance. And, the only known treatment for insulin resistance seems to be weight loss thru dieting or surgery.

Overweight Theory: A pancreas designed for a 150 lb. man simply can't make enough insulin for a 200 lb. man. Period! (see National Weight Guidelines, above)

In the past, Type I was called Juvenile Onset Diabetes. Type II was called Adult Onset Diabetes. Today, over half of new diabetic **children** are actually Type II because they're overweight. And, a large number of Type II adults end up on insulin shots if their weight doesn't come down.

BAD NEWS? Type II Diabetes is skyrocketing and mirrors our society's weight problem. The only good news is that Type II's still have some insulin. So, they can still burn glucose. That usually spares them the 'alternate fuel' problems that Type I's have.

What have you learned so far?

- Diabetes is a big problem.
- Comes in 2 Types.

- No proven cause.
- So far, no known cure.

That raises 4 big questions:

- How do you test for it?
- What are the symptoms?
- What is the treatment?
- Why do Diabetics get so sick?

———————

———

TESTING

FINGER STICK: Quick test and gives a pretty good blood sugar guesstimate.

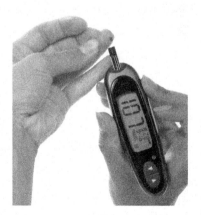

Don't forget the cost of this simple test. Initial glucose meter prices are cheap ($0-$50). But, the **test strips** may average close to $1/ day[11]. Profitability comes from using proprietary strips several times each day.

LABORATORY: Blood from a vein is often more accurate. Remember, normal fasting blood sugar is under 100. But, both these tests have the same problem. They only tell what the blood sugar is right now. What about the other 23+ hours of the day? What about last week?

AI-C: This test helps answer those questions. Red blood cells are filled with an iron protein called *Hemoglobin* and live about 120 days. Then they're broken down, recycled, and made into new red cells. During their lifetime, those cells remain completely in the blood stream. If that blood has a high sugar, it chemically changes **some** of the red cells' hemoglobin. That altered hemoglobin is abbreviated A1-C. (The full name is *Glycolated Hemoglobin A1-C)*. This test reports what % of hemoglobin has been contaminated by floating in too much sugar for the last 3 months.

Normal A1-C = less than 5.7% altered hemoglobin

Pre-Diabetic A1-C = 5.7 – 6.4 %

Diabetic A1-C = over 6.5%[12]

———————

————

SYMPTOMS

In medical school, I learned Diabetes has 3 classic symptoms – *Polyphagia, Polydipsia, and Polyuria!*...Huh??

Translated, that means Diabetics are always **hungry**, always **thirsty**, and always **peeing**! Understanding these symptoms is important.

HUNGRY: Eating supplies fuel to run your motor. Your normal fuel is glucose. But, without insulin, you can't burn it for energy. Your brain doesn't understand. "Hey, I'm weak and tired up here. Eat something & get me some energy."

THIRSTY: All body chemicals are dissolved in serum – the watery part of the blood. Each chemical has a very specific concentration. Potassium must be between 3.5 and 5.3. Acidity (pH) should be 7.35 - 7.45. Fasting glucose should be under 100. Suddenly, glucose is **500.** Quick fix? Dilute it down with lots of water. Brain says, "Just drink some more. And pull some water out of the other body cells to dilute this sugar." Extra water intake dilutes other blood chemicals out of their range. Cells giving up their water become dehydrated.

PEEING: Frequent urination is a Diabetic's 3rd symptom. The patient is drinking constantly, trying to dilute that high blood sugar. Body cells are giving up their water for the same reason. What do the kidneys think when they see all this water coming through? "We're drowning! Quick, pee it out." Result? A downhill spiral to dehydration.

DIABETIC TREATMENT

Initial treatment for Type I Diabetes and for Type II Diabetes is very different.

Type 1's usually aren't advised to lose weight. Why? Since they're burning mostly fat, they're already losing weight. Often, a lot of weight. That's not the solution for them.

Remember, TYPE I's have no insulin. To survive, they must be on insulin replacement. Originally, medical insulin came from pigs and cows. It wasn't as effective as human insulin and allergies were common.

Today, medical insulin is synthetic human insulin. There are many types, brands, and combinations. All have different peaks and durations. Their costs vary from reasonable to obscene. But, Type I Diabetes is a life sentence. Without a pancreas transplant, you're on insulin shots for life. Even with a new pancreas, you'll have the lifelong risks associated with all organ transplants.

TYPE II's have a pancreas that still makes insulin. It's just not **enough** insulin for their needs. For them, losing weight is the primary treatment. If you think weight loss is complicated, let me introduce Harvard's Dr. Frank Sacks. In 2009, he pretty much closed the book on weight loss diets. He wrote "Comparison of Weight-Loss Diets with Different Compositions of Fat, Protein, and Carbohydrates"[13]. He placed 811 overweight patients on diets containing different percentages of protein, fats, and carbohydrates. They were followed for 2 years. In the end, the only difference in weight loss was determined by the number of calories ingested. It wasn't **what** you ate, but how many **calories** you ate, that made the difference. Knowing that, the math is fairly simple. A pound of fat contains 3,500 calories. If you can eliminate 100 calories every day, you'll take off about 10 lbs. in a year.

For Type II Diabetics, if the weight doesn't come off, medications are started. We know what we want the pill to do. That's **easy**:

Make the belly stop digesting and absorbing sugar;

Make the liver stop storing sugar as Glycogen (see GLYCOGEN - above);

Make the pancreas work harder to produce more insulin;

Make body cells learn to be content with less insulin (see INSULIN RESISTANCE - above).

But, picking the **right** pill is not easy. Why? On line, The Mayo Clinic [14] lists at least 15 individual drugs. That's a lot of choices – well beyond the scope of this book.

Usually, a drug like *metformin* is tried first [15]. Why? Long track record. Generic. Inexpensive. Pretty safe (if you have good kidneys). Lowers both dietary sugar absorption and glycogen storage. Doesn't beat up that tired pancreas. Doesn't cause low blood sugar attacks.

What if weight loss and Metformin fail? All those other pills are options. But, cost, side effects, and that poor, tired pancreas can be real problems.

So, if your weight's still up. And, you've failed several kinds of pills. And, your A1-C is still climbing...

Welcome to the world of the Type I Diabetic. Here's your insulin.

———————

———

WHY DO DIABETICS GET SO SICK?

Short Term: HUNGER doesn't help. Without enough insulin, you can't burn what you're eating. THIRST doesn't help. Drinking more water just dilutes all your body chemicals out of range. PEEING doesn't help. That just leaves you very dehydrated with even more chemicals out of whack. And that's not the worst of it.

Long Term For unknown reasons, diabetes destroys blood vessels. Arteries everywhere, both large and small, form fatty deposits in their walls. That's *Atherosclerosis* or hardening of the arteries. Once hardened, they can clot off, leak, balloon out (aneurysm), or burst under pressure. The end result is the same. That artery no longer feeds the tissue it's supposed to supply. Without oxygen and nutrients, that tissue dies. Skin, heart, brain, kidneys – every organ in the body can have this tragic result.

TRANSLATING MEDICALESE

Your doctor took a History and did your Physical Exam. Your tests are back. In her office, she tells you: "It's *TTP - Thrombotic Thrombocytopenic Purpura*. We'll start you on *steroids* right away and I'll set up the *Plasma Exchange* for you." "Any questions?" she asks. You nod politely. "No, Doctor, I'm good."

Your family comes in and asks how it went. "She's starting me on steroids", you say. "Steroids," your wife says, "You mean like weight lifters? Will that help your rash?"

What happened? Your doctor just spoke to you in a foreign language – *Medicalese*. Unfortunately, you took Spanish in high school, so you haven't a clue.

This chapter has 2 purposes:

First, let's do a half dozen common illnesses. You've heard of all of them. You've used most of them in sentences. Now, you might actually know what you're talking about. Second, let's try some Medicalese. It actually makes sense – once you know the secret ground rules.

———————

———

COMMON DIAGNOSES

STREP THROAT

Short for *Acute Streptococcal Tonsillitis.* A sudden, painful, bacterial infection of the tonsils. Tonsils are part of your immune system. Your immune system fights infections. Strep Throat means strep germs overwhelmed your tonsil's ability to fight back. Most patients are children, teens, or young adults. It's rare before age 3 or after age 30.[1] Because Strep is a bacteria, antibiotics are used. But, **why** they're used is interesting. The surface of this strep germ is made of proteins that look just like the proteins on heart valve cells. Antibiotics destroy the bacteria before your body makes antibodies against it. Without antibiotics, your body **may** make antibodies that can't tell strep germs from heart cells. Result? *Rheumatic Fever (RF)* – a life-threatening complication of Strep Throat. Fortunately, it's very rare today – less than 10 cases per 100,000. [2] But, if it's a Strep Throat, you will get antibiotics. So, you've got a sore throat - ONLY 2 possibilities. It's either Strep (and needs antibiotics) or Everything-Else (and does **not** need antibiotics). How can you tell if it's strep?

3 ways:

1. Rapid Strep Test – Commercial throat swab for immediate detection of strep antigen. Test may have up to 20% False Negatives[3] (means test is negative, but patient really does have the disease). Cost? About $33. [4]
2. Throat culture - swab the throat and try to grow strep germs on a jello-plate. Test may have up to 20% False Positives[5] (test is positive but patient does not have the disease). Cost? Usually more than the Rapid Strep Test **and** takes 48 hrs.
3. Or, better still, you could examine the patient using the *Centor Criteria (Modified)*[6]. What are they, you ask?

- Is there fever over 100.4 F?
- Is there a cream cheese-like *Exudate* (covering) on the tonsils?
- Are there tender, swollen glands under the angles of the jaw?
- Is cough **Absent**?

If the patient has 3 or 4 of these, strep is likely. Under age 30, this clinical exam does as well or better than testing [7,8]. Cost? $0. Finally, **remember** - less than 10% of sore throats are strep and less than 1 in 10,000 strep throats will cause Rheumatic Fever without antibiotics.

Going on a TV game show soon?

"Jeopardy" Question: Exactly what germ causes strep throat? "Jeopardy" Answer: *Group A Beta-Hemolytic Streptococcus.*

HEARTBURN

Gastro-Esophageal Reflux Disorder – GERD for short.

Here's the deal: Your *Esophagus* (food tube) squeezes food from mouth down to stomach. The **valve** at bottom of Esophagus opens. Food is squeezed into stomach. The **valve** closes. Stomach secretes powerful *Hydrochloric Acid* to begin food breakdown. Stomach has protective lining against acid. Food tube does **not** have protective lining. As the **valve** wears out, stomach acid comes back up (refluxes) into the esophagus. Hydrochloric acid burns the lining of the esophagus causing pain.

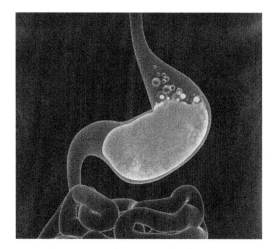

Notice that heart - as in heartburn - wasn't mentioned? Why? The esophagus lies **behind** the heart. The acid damage **feels** like burning chest pain around the heart – hence Heartburn.

- What wears out the valve: Stomach pressure from below - like pregnancy or obesity.
- Worst time for GERD: Lying down at night after eating is like 'high tide' for acid.
- Can diet make GERD worse: Yes. Acid foods (vinegar), spicy foods (peppers), fizzy sodas (fizz is carbonic **acid**), and overeating (stretches the valve) all make GERD worse.
- Can drinking alcohol effect GERD pain? (Not sure? Clean your scraped knee with alcohol – feels good, right?)
- Last, what's a *Hiatal Hernia*, and what's it got to do with GERD? That Esophagus valve becomes so loose, the top of stomach can actually pop up into the chest cavity.

Result: **Constant** reflux.

Treatment?

- Avoid things that bother your GERD.
- For single episodes, neutralize the acid with Maalox, Mylanta, or old-fashioned 1 tsp. Baking Soda in small glass of water.
- Avoid antacids containing calcium – temporary relief may be followed by **increased** acid production.
- For long term GERD, turn down the acid with H_2 Blockers (Zantac Pepcid, Axid, etc.) or with PPI's (Prilosec, Nexium, Prevacid, etc.).
- Last point. GERD is miserable. But, untreated chronic GERD may cause cancer of the esophagus. Trust me, that's more than just miserable.

Importance?

Nexium is a popular treatment for reflux. It's also Medicare's #1 drug expense.

LOW THYROID

Hypothyroidism means your thyroid gland doesn't make enough hormone. So what? Well....the brain likes to think it's in charge. Truth is, thyroid hormone regulates the entire body's metabolism. Car engines idle at different speeds. Likewise, people have different metabolic rates. Your thyroid sets the 'idle speed' of your 'engine'. Not enough hormone? Engine is sluggish or stops. Too much hormone? Like holding the gas pedal to the floor in neutral – engine overheats and explodes.

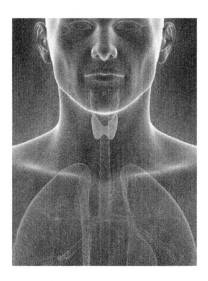

The thyroid is a butterfly shaped gland in your neck - just below your voice box. Normally, it feels smooth, pretty flat, non-tender, and has equal right and left halves. No lumps, bumps, enlargement, or pain allowed. Diabetes may be our #1 endocrine disease, but low thyroid is #2, especially in women. Symptoms are weight gain, declining memory, dry skin, coarse or thinning hair, constipation, and personality changes.

Luckily, diagnosis and treatment are both pretty straightforward. We used to start by testing various hormone levels. Today the starting point is a blood level of *TSH – Thyroid Stimulating Hormone.*[9] TSH is made in the brain. Is your brain happy with the level of thyroid hormone in the blood stream? A normal TSH usually means low thyroid is not the problem. A high TSH is the brain saying, "Hey, thyroid, wake up and make some more hormone. Let's speed things up."

Low thyroid treatment is simple – just add some hormone. Generic *levothyroxine* is a synthetic version of normal thyroid hormone. It's cheap **and** effective. (Wow, there's a first.) But, please add thyroid hormone **very** carefully. Why? Most medicines come in **milligram** dosages. Levothyroxine comes in **microgram** doses. Yes, that's **1/1000**

th of a milligram. This stuff is really potent. Doctors start at a low dose once daily. After 6 weeks, we recheck that TSH level. Still low? Add a tiny bit more hormone. When a daily dose brings the TSH back to normal, the brain, the patient, and the doctor should all be happy.

WOMEN'S #1 URINE PROBLEM

"I can't **stop** peeing! Bet I've got another *UTI*." That's short for *Urinary Tract Infection*. That's a **bacterial** infection anywhere in the urine system. Most often seen in females. Why? UTI germs are usually the same ones found in the rectum. Females have a short distance between the urine and rectal openings. Intercourse, wiping direction, exercise, tight underwear, etc. may move germs from one area to the other.

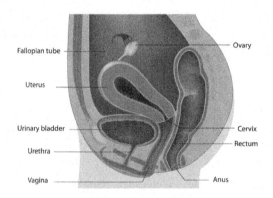

2 KINDS OF UTI's

Lower UTI's: mean infection in the bladder or urethra (tube from the bladder to the outside). Bladder infection is called *Cystitis*. Infection of the urine tube is called *Urethritis*. These two infections often occur together. With Lower UTI's, the patient is miserable but not in danger. Urine burning, frequency, urgency, and traces of blood are common. How's your doc make the diagnosis? Usually with a commercial *Urine Dipstick*.

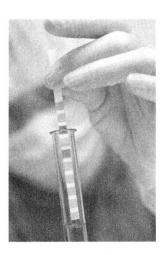

He's looking for several pads to turn color on the test strip. Blood? Usually (+). White Blood Cells? Usually (+). Most important test on the strip? A (+) nitrate test usually clinches the diagnosis. Infecting bacteria convert urine **nitrite** to **nitrate** turning that strip (+).

CAUTION #1: Red Blood Cells, White Blood Cells, and Bacteria can be normal in the vagina. **None** of these is normal in urine. That can complicate urine tests. Female patients can avoid this by a) sitting backward on the toilet, b) using one hand to open the vaginal lips, and c) collecting the urine sample using the other hand to hold the cup **midway** thru peeing. Treatment is simple as 1, 2, 3. First, give a cheap, generic antibiotic for 3-5 days. Second, add some cheap, generic *Pyridium* for 1-2 days (turns urine bright orange and works like novacaine to stop symptoms). And third, drink lots of fluids to flush things through.

CAUTION #2: If the patient also has a vaginal discharge, this may be an *STD (Sexually Transmitted Disease)*. Most ER docs consider all women sexually active and that STD's are always possible – even if the patient denies both.

Upper UTI's - a kidney infection. This one's serious. Why? Kidneys filter your blood. An infected 'filter' could infect your whole blood stream. And, these patients are really sick – high fever, shaking chills, tender kidney(s), and even vomiting. PLUS, they may have all those miserable Lower UTI symptoms as well. These patients are often admitted for *I.V.* antibiotics for a day or so.

———————

———

MEN'S #1 URINE PROBLEM

"I can't **start** peeing!" Why? Probably an enlarged prostate. (Admit it guys, you're not real sure what a prostate is, are you?)

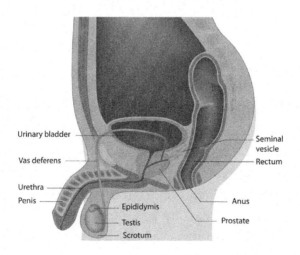

It's in front of the rectum and just below the bladder. It has a central hole to pee through. When you're young it works pretty well and is about the size of a walnut.

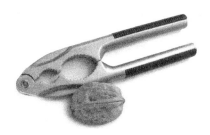

SIZE OF NORMAL PROSTATE

Prostate: Good News? Bad News? The good news is twofold. Unlike women, the tip of the penis is **not** near the anus. So, men rarely get bladder infections. And, the prostate is a great help making sexual secretions. (Remember that. Prostate infections may be sexually transmitted.) Unfortunately, the bad news is also twofold – *BPH* and *Prostate cancer*: **BPH** is short for ***Benign Prostatic Hypertrophy*** - prostate enlargement. Well, "benign" is good because it's not cancer. But, enlargement is not good.

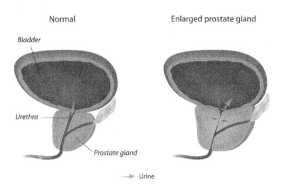

Benign Prostatic Hyperplasia

Normal   Enlarged prostate gland

Bladder

Urethra

Prostate gland

Urine

47

As the entire prostate gets bigger the hole to pee through gets smaller. Symptoms? Ask any man over 60. *Frequency* because bladder can't completely empty through that small hole. *Urgency* because the bladder never fully empties and needs to go again right now. *Hesitancy* because starting urine through that small opening requires straining. *Nocturia* because those daily symptoms go on all night. Various medications may help temporarily. But, usually it's a surgeon who cuts, Roto-Rooters, or lasers out the prostate to open urine flow again. How large can the prostate get? As big as a LEMON!

Prostate Cancer is the #1 major organ cancer in men – about 200,000 cases per year[10]. It's also the #2 cause of cancer death in men – about 29,000 per year[11]. But, those 2 facts are the ONLY simple information about this disease. Why?[12]

Symptoms: Many localized cancers cause NO symptoms and may grow slowly. When symptoms develop they may be identical to symptoms of prostate enlargement or infection.

WARNING: blood in urine or sexual secretions is very suspicious. PSA Screening: *PSA* is short for *Prostate Specific Antigen* – a protein from the prostate that can be tested in the blood. It goes up in prostate cancer. **But**, PSA results vary by patient age, race, medications, infections, prostate size, etc.

Clinical *DRE* Screening: **DRE** means **D**igital **R**ectal **E**xam. Remember, the prostate's right in front of the rectum. Feeling thru the rectal wall, a doctor's finger may detect enlargement, lumps, or tenderness.

Screening Errors: Both PSA and DRE can have false positive and false negative results. Needle Biopsy: Identifies slow vs. fast growing prostate cancers. This helps guide therapy. But, infection, bleeding, and pain after biopsy are significant drawbacks.[13] "Dying **from** Prostate Cancer" and "Dying **with** Prostate Cancer" are very different. The 40 year old needs aggressive treatment right now to save his life. An 80 year old will probably die from something else before his prostate cancer becomes important.

PROBLEM? It's often hard to sort out which category you're in.

LARGE INTESTINE PROBLEMS (SIMPLIFIED)

Diverticulitis, Appendicitis, Hemorrhoids, and Colon Cancer. All these are **far** more common in America than 3rd World Countries. And, they're all *Large Intestine* problems.

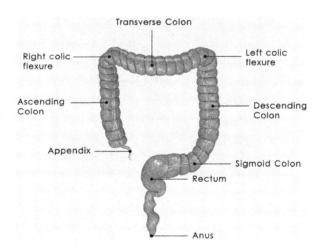

Your Large Intestine has 2 important functions: to absorb water from the diet and to store stool until the next bowel movement. Longer storage means more water is absorbed. That causes harder stools and constipation, which increases pressure inside bowel. Let's look at each diagnosis.

Diverticulitis: tiny out-pouchings of the Large Intestine, probably from stool pressure. Rare before age 40, almost universal by age 90. May cause no symptoms. But, may cause bleeding, become obstructed, or burst (life-threatening).

Appendicitis: Obstruction of the cavity of the appendix, often from backed up stool. Common: about 5% of Americans especially in their teens and 20's.The obstruction causes infection. Without treatment the appendix will swell and burst. Dangerous? **50%** death rate without surgery and antibiotics.

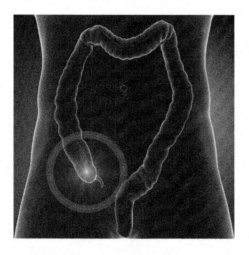

Hemorrhoids: this one's easy. Picture the worst varicose leg veins you've seen. Twisty, blue, bulging veins, right? Well, Hemorrhoids are really just *Varicose Veins* of your butt. All veins are thin walled blood vessels returning blood to the heart. Pressure on a vein blocks its flow making it bulge out. If you don't believe it's that simple, ask any 9 month pregnant woman.

Anal Disorders

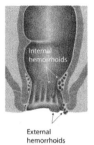 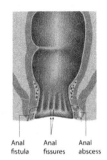

External
hemorrhoids

Anal   Anal   Anal
fistula   fissures   abscess

If the bulging vein is **inside** the anus, hard stool scrapes the hemorrhoid causing bleeding. That's an *Internal Hemorrhoid*. A bulging vein **outside** the anus itches and burns. That's an *External Hemorrhoid*. If blood in an External Hemorrhoid **clots**? Well, you'll recall the pain long after a surgeon numbs it and removes the clot.

Colon Cancer: For men and women, colorectal cancer is our #2 cause of cancer deaths[14]. Is constipation a risk factor? Sorry, the jury's still out on that one. There are good journal articles on both sides.[15,16,17] Meanwhile, simply adding more fiber and water to our diet is easy and cheap. It also mimics 3rd world diets where colon problems are uncommon. Why not try it?

———————

———

MEDICALESE: Remember page 1 of this chapter? That patient had TTP – **Thrombotic Thrombocytopenic Purpura**. Now that's really Medicalese. Below is a list of medical prefixes, suffixes, and abbreviations. They're often linked together. So, *Thrombo* anything means a blood clot. *Cyto* means a cell. *Penic* means too few. And, *Purpura* means a purple rash from bleeding.

Put it all together. Clotting is good when you're bleeding. Clotting is BAD when you're not bleeding. So, TTP means something made this patient start clotting **all over** (Thrombotic). That process used up all her clotting cells (Thrombo – Cyto – Penic). Now, she's bleeding **all over**. The purple rash (Purpura) means she's even bleeding under her skin. A horrendous disease? Absolutely, but now at least you can understand it.

MEDICAL PREFIXES AND SUFFIXES

arthro ... joint

cardio ... heart

colo ... colon (large intestine)

cranio ... head or toward the head

cyto ... cell

derm ... skin

dorso or *dorsal* ... back of the body

ectomy ... surgeon removes something

emia ... some quantity of something in the blood

enia ... too little of something in the blood

gastro ... stomach

hypo ... too little or too few

hyper ... too much or too many

itis ... inflamed or infected

larygo ... voice box

myo ... muscle

nephro ... kidney

neuro ... brain, spinal cord, nerves

oto ... ear

otomy ... surgeon opens something

pharyngo ... throat

pulmo ... lung

purpur ... purple rash like bruising
rhino ... nose
syno ... lining of a joint
teno ... tendon
thrombo ... clot
ventro or *ventral* ... front of the body

ORTHOPEDICS:
THE FRAMEWORK THAT HOLDS YOU TOGETHER

Raise your hand if you've never broken a bone in your entire life. You're a minority. At some time, most of us break something. Maybe just a finger or toe. Remember when you ran barefoot through the house? Caught that toe on the leg of the coffee table. CRACK. Toe crooked. Doctor numbed it. Set it straight. Taped two toes together for a couple weeks. Hurt like Hell! OK, now you remember.

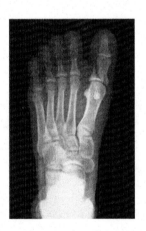

(Broken Big Toe)

For fingers and toes, your family doc probably did the fix. For everything bigger, an *Orthopedist* got the call. Their specialty, *Orthopedics,* was first named for *Ortho* meaning **to straighten** and *Peds* meaning **children**. Straightening children's injured or diseased limbs was their original job.

Definition: Orthopedics – medical specialty diagnosing and treating injuries and diseases of the musculoskeletal system. OK, you knew they handled injuries. What diseases could they handle? How about *Septic Arthritis* (infected joint). Or maybe the disease is *Osteosarcoma* (a bad bone cancer). Even immune diseases like *Rheumatoid Arthritis* may need an orthopedist's help.

Now, I want you to remember **three** numbers: **7**, **6**, and **5**. Why? Because your musculoskeletal system has **7** parts. It's prone to **6** common injuries. And, when any part becomes *Inflamed* you get **5** symptoms.

Anatomy first. Let's start with those **7 PARTS**:

Bones – the body's rigid framework. Children's x-rays show a thin, dark horizontal line across the bone. This is called the *Epiphysis* or growth line. It allows the bone to lengthen with age. When growth is completed, the line turns to white, solid bone and disappears. (Compare child an adult bone x-rays below)

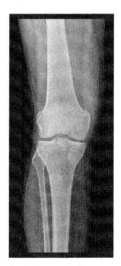 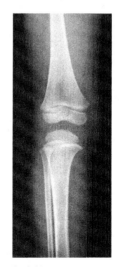

Adult's Knee X-ray   **Child's Knee X-ray**

Joints – space between two bone ends

Cartilage – slippery pad covering bone ends to prevent grinding

Ligaments – bands of tissue holding bones together at a joint

Tendons – bands of tissue holding muscles to bones

Muscles – contractile tissue that pulls tendons to move bones

Bursa – water balloons to cushion bony angles (like hip, knee, and shoulder)

Only bones and joints, can be seen on x-ray (see above). The rest all show up as gray.

Why? Let's talk about x-rays. Imagine x-ray film as **white**. It turns **black** when an x-ray beam hits it. With only air in its path, the beam gets thru, and the film turns black. If we try to x-ray through a steel plate, **no** radiation gets to the film. Result? The film stays white.

Now, x-rays of humans. People's x-rays have only have 3 shades – White, Black, and Gray. So, bones look white – very little radiation got thru to that white film. Lungs are air-filled so most of the radiation got thru. They look black. Everything else is *Soft Tissue*. Some radiation got thru that soft tissue and turned the film **gray**. Problem: all soft tissues are the **same** gray on x-ray. So, cartilage, ligaments, tendons, muscles, and organs all look gray. No details can be seen.

Black = air around hand

White = all hand bones

Gray = all other hand tissues

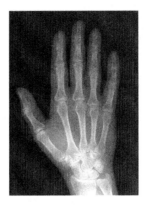

———————

———

Now, how about those **6 INJURIES**? You do remember there were 6 orthopedic injuries, right?

Contusion (Bruise) – broken *Capillaries* (tiny blood vessels) leak under the skin

Hematoma (Blood Blister) – broken blood vessel under the skin forms a puddle of blood

Fracture (Break) – **any** broken bone is a fracture

Strain (with a '**t**') – stretching or tearing of a **tendon** or muscle

Sprain – stretched or torn **ligaments** holding bones together

Dislocation – end of bone pops out of joint

———————

———

OK, you got the 7 parts and the 6 injuries. Now, the **5 SIGNS OF INFLAMMATION**. **Definition:** Inflammation is a normal body response to injury or infection. It starts our *Fight and Heal* reaction. The 5 classic symptoms are:

Red - Extra blood flow is opened to the area.

Hot – That extra blood flow increases local heat.

Swollen - Platelets and clotting chemicals rush to stop bleeding. White blood cells sneak out into tissues to hunt down invaders and begin cleanup.

Painful - Limits the use of the area, allowing it to rest.

Won't work– Until healing is complete, skin, muscle, bone, tendon, etc. can't perform normally.

One last note on inflammation. Any medical term ending in **itis** means it's inflammation. So, tendon**itis** is an inflamed tendon. Burs**itis** is an inflamed bursa, and so on.

———————

———

So, now you know the 7 Musculoskeletal Parts, 6 Injuries, and 5 Signs of Inflammation. You know Orthopedists treat all that. How do they spend most of their time? Treating 'The BIG 5':

FRACTURES

Definition: All broken bones are fractures. But, there are **many** different kinds of fractures: *Simple* (bone breaks into 2 pieces) *Comminuted* (several pieces) *Angulated or Displaced* (bone pieces in poor position) *Hairline* (barely visible) *Incomplete* (part way thru bone) *Complete* (all the way thru) *Green-stick* (bent or buckled in kids) *Closed* (skin intact over the fracture) *Compound* (fracture open thru the skin – **BAD** and likely to get infected!)

For adults, the most common large bone fractures are wrists and hips. In kids, it's collar bones and wrists.

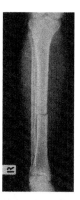

Simple Fracture Lower Leg:

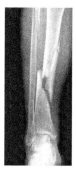

Comminuted Fracture Lower Leg

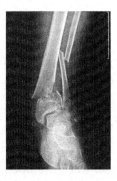

Angulated Fracture Lower Leg

————————

———

SHOULDER PAIN

Anatomy: The shoulder includes the *Scapula* (shoulder blade), the *Clavicle* (collar bone), the *Humerus* (upper arm bone), and all their attachments.

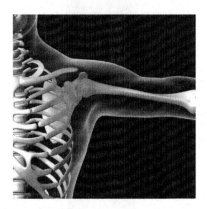

Use your right hand to scratch the back of your head. Now scratch your left shoulder. Next, scratch your low back. Finally, wave your hand overhead like a kid signaling a teacher. Yes, the shoulder has the greatest range of motion of any joint in your body. That's the good news. The bad news? Most joints are held together by strong ligaments – 5 for an ankle, 4 for a knee, etc. Ligaments keep those joints stable, but limit their motion. Shoulders are the opposite. The shoulder blade has 1 muscle on the front and 3 muscles on its back. Each muscle has a tendon. Those 4 tendons wrap around the shoulder joint like a 'cuff', holding it together. That's the *Rotator Cuff.* Unlike ligaments, the muscles and tendons are flexible. That gives the shoulder its great range of motion.

Rotator Cuff Muscles

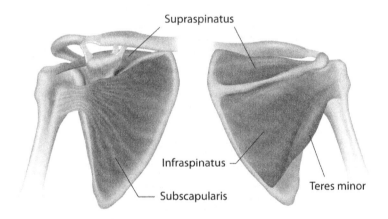

Shoulder Blade - Front view   **Shoulder Blade – Back View**

Why are those tendons bad news? The shoulder's wide range of motion often inflames, tears, or wears out that Rotator Cuff holding it together. That's significant pain for the patient, and more business for the orthopedic surgeon. More bad news? The shoulder is the #1 large joint dislocation. Each episode tears part of that rotator cuff. That weakens the joint, making the next dislocation more likely. Surgery is often needed after several episodes.

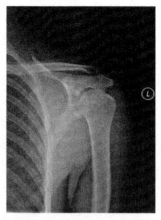

NORMAL SHOULDER

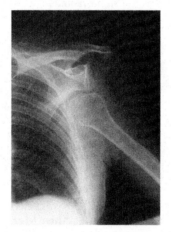

DISLOCATED SHOULDER

SPINE PAIN

Anatomy: A curved column of 25 bones that hold us upright. The *Spinal Cord* lies in a tunnel at the **back** of the column. The **rest** of the body lies in **front** of the spinal column. The spine is divided into 4 regions:

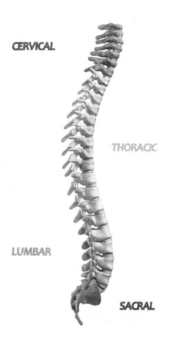

CERVICAL SPINE (neck) – the top 7 *vertebrae* (bones) of the column. It's the back of the neck, and normally hollowed out.

THORACIC SPINE (chest)– the next 12 vertebrae of the column. It's the back of the chest and it's rounded backwards.

LUMBAR SPINE (low back)– the 5 vertebrae between the chest and the waist. Like the neck, it's concave when seen from the side.

SACRAL SPINE – (butt) The base of the spinal column from waist to tailbone (*Coccyx*). It really has 5 bones. (They're all fused so we'll treat them as one.)

What spine areas cause the most problems? The neck and the low back:

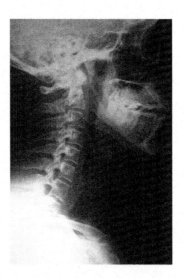

X-ray CERVICAL SPINE – Side View

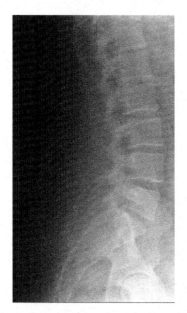

X-ray LUMBAR SPINE – Side View

So, the Spine is a complex column of bones. Has 4 separate curves to give it flexibility. Multiple ligaments, tendons, and muscles hold it all together. So, what's the big deal? **Pain**, that's the big deal! Low Back

Pain is our #1 cause of injury disability. It's probably the #1 reason patients see a doctor over their lifetime. Neck strains and sprains from whiplash injury are a big cause of lawsuits. Everybody seems to have a *Slipped Disc* or *Pinched Nerve,* whatever they are. Let's look at these one at a time.

Low Back Pain – Animals walking on all fours do much better than human beings. Standing erect requires our lower spine (Lumbar) to be concave. It helps maintain our center of balance. It also crimps the spine and spinal cord at the waist. Next trip to the zoo, take a look at the gorilla. Spends most of his day on all fours and has a nice FLAT lumbar spine. It only becomes concave in the moments when he stands upright. Now watch the next 9-month-pregnant woman you see. She's wincing and holding her low back, right? Why? If she doesn't lean **backward** the baby's weight will make her fall **forward**. Obesity? Same problem. But, increasing that lumbar hollow curve has a price. It shortens the muscles in the low back. That's fine until you bend over to tie your shoe. Remember the injury name for overstretched muscles and tendons? It's called Strain. **Diagnosis**: *Acute Low Back Pain Secondary to Lumbar Strain.* Does this patient need an x-ray? **NO!** Remember, **all** soft tissues are the same shade of gray on x-ray. Normal, strained, and sprained soft tissues all look the same. "But", you say, "bones are white and might show a fracture"... Do you really think you broke your back bending to tie your shoes?

Slipped Disc – Find two 4" building blocks like kids play with. Stack them one on top of the other - like vertebrae. Two problems – not much range of motion and no shock absorber in case of fall. Now, put a nice, soft, creme-filled donut between the blocks. Wiggle the stack. Range of motion's better, right? If you dropped the stack, the donut could cushion some of the force, right?

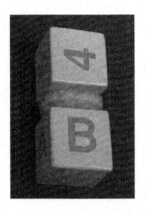 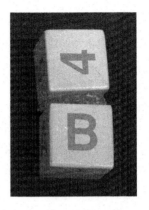

NORMAL SPINE   AGING SPINE

All vertebrae are separated by *Intervertebral Discs.* Like donuts, the discs are firm on the outside (*Annulus Fibrosis)* and creme-like on the inside (*Nucleus Pulposus).* Unfortunately, like donuts, our discs don't improve with age. They get stale, crumble down, and wear out. That's called *Degenerative Disc Disease.*

DISC DEGENERATION

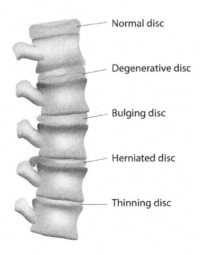

— Normal disc

— Degenerative disc

— Bulging disc

— Herniated disc

— Thinning disc

Now, push down hard on the top building block. What happens? The creme center squirts **out** of the donut. In the spine, the only way **out** is back and to the side. What's "back and to the side"? The nerves coming off the spinal cord. **Diagnosis**: *Acute Herniated Intervertebral Disc with Nerve Root Compression.* In English, that's a slipped disc and a pinched nerve. It really hurts. And, it really hurts in **2** places – where the nerve is pinched **AND** all along the course of that nerve.

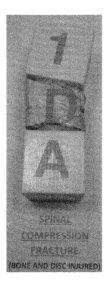

Compression Fracture – as bones thin with age, a simple fall on your butt may squash a vertebra, a *Compression Fracture.*

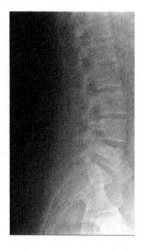 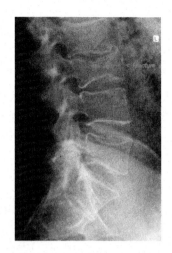

NORMAL LUMBAR SPINE   **BROKEN LUMBAR SPINE**

When does Low Back Pain become a true Emergency? E.R. docs usually look for **Red Flags:**

1. Did the patient lose control of bowels or bladder?
2. Is there paralysis or weakness in all or part of a lower extremity?
3. Was the mechanism of injury enough to break bones?
4. Did the patient **ever** have cancer **anywhere?**

Whiplash Injury – You're the right front passenger in a car going 65 mph. You're wearing your lap and shoulder seat belts. Tractor trailer pulls directly across in front of your car. CRASH! Your vehicle goes from 65 mph to 0 mph almost immediately. Your seat belt pretty much stops your body when the car stops. Ah, but your head's not restrained. It continues to travel straight ahead at 65 mph until your neck stops it. That means all the bones, ligaments, tendons, and muscles in your neck get stretched **forward** to their max. Then for good measure, your head rebounds as far **backward** as it can go. That's until it smacks into the headrest. Any question why your neck doesn't move right the next day? Any question why you have a headache?

The last point about back pain is surgery. The true emergencies above require surgery. But, most studies show that surgery done explicitly for pain relief only helps about half the patients.

KNEE JOINT

(Front view/ Kneecap removed)

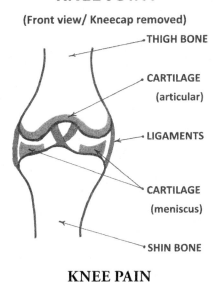

THIGH BONE

CARTILAGE
(articular)

LIGAMENTS

CARTILAGE
(meniscus)

SHIN BONE

KNEE PAIN

Definition: Hinge-type joint at the middle of the lower extremity. BONES: Each knee has 3 bones: the *Femur* (thigh bone), the *Tibia* (shin bone), and the *Patella* (knee cap). The femur and tibia bear the weight. The patella acts like a pulley to help thigh muscles straighten the lower leg.

LIGAMENTS: 4 tough ligaments hold the knee together. Those ligaments **only** allow the knee to bend and straighten – like a hinge. Normal knees have **no** rotation and **no** buckling from side to side.

CARTILAGE: 3 slippery cartilages protect the knee. The end of the thigh bone is covered by *Articular Cartilage.* This is slippery, smooth and helps range of motion. Each of the other 2 cartilages is a *Meniscus* (Greek for Moon). They're crescent shaped pads that keep the thigh bone and shin bone from banging together.

BURSA: The *Pre-patellar Bursa* is a water balloon in front of the knee cap. It cushions the thigh muscle's tendon as it slides back and forth over the knee cap (*Patella*).

INJURY: Remember knees are **strickly** hinge joints. Any attempt to go bow-legged, knock-kneed, or rotate **must** tear something. Usually, it's one of the 4 ligaments that tears. Without their stability, cartilage tears, or grinds down over time.

ARTHRITIS: Inflammation of a joint. In the knee, obesity and abnormal motion gradually destroy protective cartilage. That inflames the joint. Lots of pain makes knees our #1 joint replacement. And, arthritis is the #1 cause.

EXERCISE: Strong leg muscles can stabilize a knee even when ligaments and cartilage are wearing out. Unfortunately, most leg exercises actually make knees worse. Don't believe it? Pedal your bike a mile or so. How many times did those pedals grind your knees up and down? Deep knee bends with weights? Great, let's squash those cartilages while we're grinding them. Running? How many concussive steps per mile? Some isometric exercises can strengthen the knee without wearing it out. If your doc OK's your ligaments, "The Chair" is one to try. Too easy you say? Assume the position. Great. Now, just stay there for a minute or two. Still too easy?

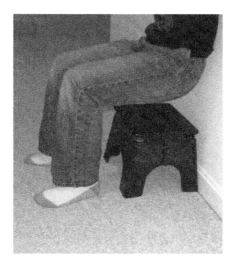

(The little stool's for safety - when your thigh
muscles get too tired to stand up!)

HAND PAIN

This is often caused by *Carpal Tunnel Syndrome.* **Definition:** Hand
pain and numbness from *Median Nerve* compression at the wrist. Roll
up your sleeve. Hold your hand out, palm up. Now, wiggle your fingers.
See the muscles moving in your forearm? See the tendons moving at
the wrist? Muscle contracts, pulls its tendon, tendon pulls its bone,
finger wiggles. At the wrist, all those tendons pass through a tough,
fibrous tunnel - the *Carpal Tunnel.* So far, so good. No pain, right?
Unfortunately, the delicate Median Nerve also runs thru the tunnel.
That nerve supplies pain fibers for the palm aspect of the thumb and
the next 2 ½ fingers.

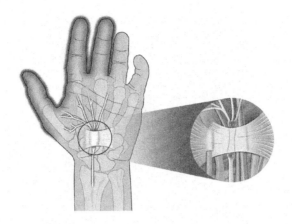

**Median Nerve passing through
Carpal Tunnel and out to fingers.**

Imagine you're playing the piano. Those tendons are sliding back and forth like crazy. Each movement also rubs that poor median nerve. Even worse, how about a computer keyboard? Why worse? With typing, the wrists are held cocked up. That crimps the tunnel and increases friction. Chronic wear and tear leads to inflammation which leads to **Pain**.

Treatment is 3 stages:

Ice bag, rest, and NSAID pills (like naproxen) for the inflammation.

Perhaps a daily wrist splint (Yes, it hurts more at night, but the injury is during the day).

Not better in 2 months? Steroid (cortisone) shot often gives a couple months' relief.

By 1 year over 75% of patients require surgery.[1]

MEDICATIONS:
GENERICS, ANALGESICS, ANTIBIOTICS, VACCINES, ETC.

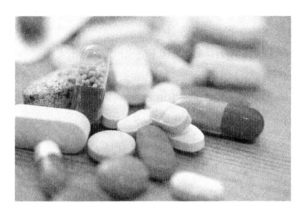

BRAND NAME vs. GENERIC DRUGS –
Worth the price difference?

Much research and many studies show no significant difference between brand name and generic medication.[1,2] No difference, that is, except a **huge** cost.

Here's how it works: A drug company thinks they have a new blockbuster. Quick, give it a catchy name and patent it. That protects the discovery – and brand name – for 20 years. After that, other companies can make the drug in generic form. But, the clock started at patent filing. The company still needs clinical testing, FDA approval, and marketing before the first sale. That takes years off that 20 year patent protection.

Here are some common over-the-counter medicines. Compare the cost of the brand name with the generic[3]. Surprised?

Pain and Fever (bottle of 24)

1. *Tylenol 500 mg* - $3.68 (acetaminophen 500 mg - $1.96)
2. *Motrin 200 mg* - $2.08 (ibuprofen 200 mg - $0.88 for 40 pills)
3. *Advil 200 mg* - $3.48 (ibuprofen 200 mg - $0.88 for 40 pills)
4. *Aleve 220 mg* - $3.87 (naproxen 220 mg - $2.58)

Acid Reflux/ Heartburn/ G.E.R.D (30 day supply at one pill per day)

1. *Prilosec 20 mg* - $16.84 (omeprazole 20 mg - $9.13) 2. *Prevacid 15 mg* - $20.88 (lansoprazole 15 mg - $13.80)[3]

OK, so why do doctors write so many brand name prescriptions? 2 clever reasons.

- First, many prescription pads come preprinted with the words "Dispense as Written" on them. That means a Pharmacist cannot substitute a generic.
- Read any prescription brand name out loud. Are you more likely to remember brand name antibiotic *Augmentin* or amoxicillin/clavulanate? The tranquilizer *Xanax* or generic alprazolam? Patient has diarrhea – *Lomotil* or diphenoxylate/atropine? Which is quicker to write when your waiting room is swamped with patients?

My proposal to help balance the Federal budget – and yours:

When a drug patent expires, **all** prescriptions for the drug will be filled with a generic. Two exceptions:

a) New research proves the brand name is clinically better or safer. (Ask your pharmacist.)

b) Patient pays the price difference. (Don't hold your breath!)

PAIN MEDICATIONS

Q: How many types of pain medication exist on planet Earth?

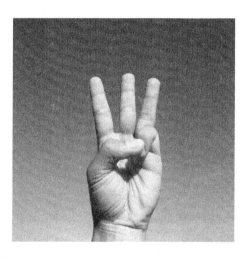

A: Did you hold up 3 fingers? You win!

"What?" "Are you crazy?" "There must be hundreds of medicines for pain!" You're right. There are hundreds of pain medicines. But, they all fall into **3** types:

Tylenol (generic - acetaminophen): Basic over-the-counter analgesic for mild to moderate pain. Works somehow, somewhere in the brain. Very safe in small children, but overdoses in adults may seriously damage the liver.

NSAID's (**N**on-**S**teroidal **A**nti-**I**nflammatory **D**rugs): *Cortisone* is a steroid and was the first anti-inflammation drug. Way too many side effects! The second anti-inflammation drug was... *Aspirin*, a **non**-steroid drug. Good, but still had lots of side effects with chronic use. Next came all the other NSAID's out there: *Advil (*ibuprofen*), Motrin* (also ibuprofen), *Aleve* (naproxen), *Celebrex* (celecoxib), etc. Pain is often caused by inflammation, so **anti**-inflammation drugs make sense. Main concerns are stomach bleeding and kidney effects.

Narcotics, from an ancient Greek word meaning "to make numb" (also called *Opioids*).When it comes to pain, those Greeks really knew their stuff. **All** narcotics target specific receptors in the brain. Good news? The best pain relief known. Bad news? Side effects, like can't think, can't drive, can't stay awake, can't work, can't pee, and can't poop. **Worst** news? All narcotics, regardless of type or dose, are addictive. Addiction means two things:

1. **Tolerance**: Your brain adapts to overcome the sedative effect of the narcotic. So, you're going to need ever-higher doses to keep getting the same effect.

2. **Withdrawal**: When taking narcotics, all systems speed up to overcome sedation. Coming off narcotics, all systems are still at high speed, without that narcotic emergency brake. Nausea, vomiting, diarrhea, cramps, sweats, rapid pulse, high blood pressure, and of course, intense drug craving. **Horrendous** news? Too much narcotic makes you forget everything, including forgetting to breathe.

DRUG ABUSE AND ADDICTION

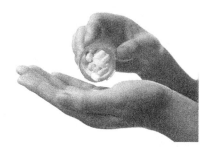

Sorry folks, IV heroin, crack cocaine, and methamphetamine aren't America's top drug problems. Alcohol is by far #1. **But**, #2 is probably medication drug abuse. That's right, abuse of doctor's prescriptions for "controlled" medications is rampant. Why is this a bigger problem than street drugs? Drug dealers are meaner, better armed, and less understanding than your doctor or pharmacist. Out at dinner with friends? It's OK to take a prescribed pill before eating. Rolling up your sleeve to shoot IV heroin? Probably not a good idea. Fainting from a medication gets you sympathy. Buying 'meth' gets you a court date.

On the street, what are the top sellers? In my practice, they're the potent narcotic Percocet (oxycodone + Tylenol) and the dreadful tranquilizer Xanax (alprazolam). Xanax's rapid onset and short duration [4] make it easily addictive. Yet it "does not appear superior to other benzodiazipines (tranquilizers like Valium)...but is more often associated with...abuse and overdose." [5]

How can these prescription drugs lead to our heroin epidemic? Simple. Doctor prescribes short term narcotic for non-cancer pain. Patient abuses the dosage and frequency. Patient gets hooked - narcotic addiction. Doctor declines a renewal. Patient tries to buy more pills on the street. Very expensive. Heroin may cost as little as $10. Just roll up your sleeve…

———————

——

FEVER

By fever, I don't mean your body temperature frying in the desert, freezing in the Arctic, or soaring past 105 from a cocaine overdose. I mean little 4 year old Johnnie has a cold and his temperature is 104 F at 9 pm. You had the same cold 10 days ago. Your temperature was only 99.9 F. He's miserable. Neither of you will sleep tonight if you don't do something. Time for some "Myth Busters".

Fever is a normal body response to infection - miserable but not dangerous. The brain increases metabolism for the fight. That includes raising body temperature. Johnnie's infection **might** be dangerous, but his fever is not.

Why was your temperature 99.9 F, yet your child's is 104? Same reason Johnnie can't do calculus yet. His brain is simply too immature to do precise work.

Please **don't** stick him in cold water – he's already miserable.

Please **do** give him some pediatric Tylenol or Children's Motrin. Both will reset his brain's 'thermostat' to a more comfortable level for a few hours

No, one isn't better than the other – Tylenol and Motrin both work well for fever.

No, don't alternate the two – doesn't work any better and costs more.

No, don't invest in gimmicky thermometers: rectal for small children, oral for everyone else.

Yes, Mom, your hand on his forehead **is** pretty good. Is it time for his next Tylenol dose?

———————

———

ANTIBIOTIC RESISTANCE

Physicians only get half the blame for this one. You patients absolutely **love** antibiotics. It's like some violent computer game. Nasty invaders from somewhere attack our unsuspecting hero (or heroine). Home defenses aren't working fast enough. Sound the bugle of modern medicine. "Here comes the Antibiotics. Death to the invaders."

Let's review a bit. Fact #1. Two kinds of germs cause most human infections, viruses and bacteria. The vast majority of infections are viral. Fact #2. Antibiotics only kill bacteria. They do **not** kill viruses. Fact #3. Giving antibiotics for viral infections **causes** antibiotic resistance. Fact #4. Let's say you take an antibiotic for a viral infection, "Just to be safe". What happens? The antibiotic does **nothing** for your viral infection. But, that antibiotic **does** kill every single bacteria it can, good or bad. Fact #5. Now, the **only** bacteria left in your body are the ones **resistant** to that antibiotic. Fact #6. Without competition, those remaining bacteria can reproduce widely.

Why do doctors prescribe antibiotics when they shouldn't? Two diagnoses seem to be the biggest offenders: *Sinusitis* and *Bronchitis*. In otherwise normal patients these conditions are usually caused by virus colds or allergies, **not** bacteria. True bacterial sinusitis is uncommon and painful. Likewise, bacterial bronchitis most always occurs in patients with pre-existing lung disease like Asthma, COPD, or Emphysema. (see "Lungs")

Just a thought: Instead of, "Hey Doc, where's my antibiotic?", how about, "Do I really need an antibiotic now?" or "Would you take one?"

History lesson: Methicillin was a great antibiotic for staph germs, until **MRSA** developed. What's MRSA? **M**ethicillin **R**esistant **S**taphylococcus **A**ureus. Oops, guess we overused that drug. Heard about **VRSA** yet? VRSA is a MRSA germ that's now also resistant to the antibiotic Vancomycin. Why's that important? Vancomycin was the drug we used to give for MRSA infections.

PRESCRIPTION DRUG ADS ON TV

Hope you're sitting down. Bad news: TV medication ads may be misleading.

From a great journal article: "Although only about one in ten major claims made in these television drug ads were judged to be demonstrably false, more than half were found to be misleading."[6]

Need an example? A brand name blood thinner, boasts 35% fewer strokes compared to the old time blood thinner for atrial fibrillation. True. On the old drug, 1.71% of fibrillation patients had a stroke. On the new, more expensive drug **only** 1.11% of those patients had a stroke. Yes, 1.11 **is** 35% less than 1.71, but....am I the only one feeling misled? [7] Oh, one more thing, if you're on a blood thinner and start to bleed, the old drug has an antidote. The new drug also got an antidote—after a $650 million lawsuit!

AMERICAN DRUG PRICES

Studies have shown that Americans may pay more for the same medication than patients in other countries. This is true even when the medication is made in the U.S.A. by an American pharmaceutical company. Those companies often rank near the top of the Fortune 500 for profitably (over 15% return on investment).[8]

Drug companies defend their high prices, blaming the high cost of research to find new and better drugs. Unfortunately, that doesn't seem to be the case. A 2012 medical journal article said, "Pharmaceutical research and development (R&D) turns out mostly minor variations on existing drugs."[9] In reviewing that article, Alexander Eichler wrote, "The authors go on to state that for every dollar pharmaceutical companies spend on basic research, $19 goes toward promotion and marketing."[10] That "British Medical Journal" article was not the first to report marketing budgets in excess of Research and Development spending. "The Cost of Pushing Pills: a New Estimate of Pharmaceutical Expenditures in the U.S." was published in 2008.[11]

Last, remember those three new blood thinners advertised on TV? (see "TV Prescription Drug Ads" - above) Each of them is about **80 times** the monthly cost of the old drug.[12]

VACCINES

To understand Vaccines, you need to meet your 'Department of Defense' – the Immune System.

Immunity: Complex body defenses against 'foreign invaders'.

Germs: Bacteria and viruses that gain entry into your body. They attack, enter human cells, and destroy them. With time, the body catalogs each new germ, including its surface proteins.

Antigen: Specific, recognizable, surface proteins of a germ, much like a fingerprint.

Antibody: A protein we manufacture to interlock with a germ's antigen and neutralize it, like a nut on a bolt.

Immune Memory: The body stores a small sample of every antibody it's ever made. It's available for 'mass production' if that germ ever comes back.

Vaccines: Dead or inactive germs injected to trigger immunity.

Vaccinations: Some infections move too quickly for our usual antibody response. Vaccinations expose the body to a germ's antigens **before** any infection. That way the exact antibody blueprint is ready if that germ does invade.

Active Immunization: The patient is exposed to the killed or inactivated germ (the Antigen) and builds his own antibodies.

Passive Immunization: The infected patient is given the specific needed Antibodies collected from another patient who survived the infection. (Often called Anti-Serum).

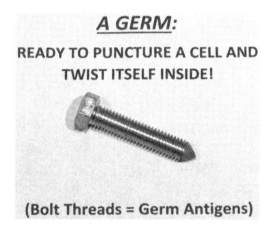

A GERM:

READY TO PUNCTURE A CELL AND TWIST ITSELF INSIDE!

(Bolt Threads = Germ Antigens)

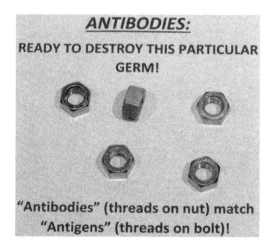

ANTIBODIES:

READY TO DESTROY THIS PARTICULAR GERM!

"Antibodies" (threads on nut) match "Antigens" (threads on bolt)!

NEW VACCINE:

INACTIVE GERMS READY TO TRIGGER ANTIBODY PRODUCTION.

Vaccine Germs are Harmless
(Cut Short and No Point)

But, Germ Antigens (the threads)
are Unchanged.

NEW ANTIBODIES –

TRIGGERED BY THE VACCINE!

Neutralize the vaccine "germs" and
stand ready for real germ attack!

ANTIGEN-ANTIBODY REACTION:

GERM IS NEUTRALIZED!

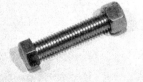

(Point is Gone and Threads are Blocked)

YOUR LUNGS: JUST TAKE SOME NICE, DEEP BREATHS

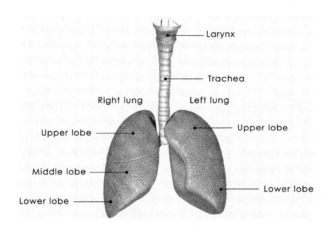

JOB DESCRIPTION FOR LUNGS: Breathe. Simple, right? Hmm…

Definition: Breathing is working to inhale, followed by relaxing to exhale.

HOW OFTEN DO WE BREATHE? That's easy. Sitting here reading, you're inhaling and exhaling 15-20 times a minute. That rate doubles or triples with exercise or stress.

HOW MUCH DO WE BREATHE? While relaxed, each breath moves about a half quart of air in and out. Maximum breathing can move over **4 quarts** of air in and out.

HOW DO WE BREATHE? Unlike solids, gas molecules bounce around in their container. That bouncing causes pressure. More bouncing molecules = more pressure. High pressure areas try to bounce into low pressure areas to equalize. **Definition:** *Atmospheric Pressure* is the weight of the Earth's air pressing down on us. At sea level, that's about 14.7 pounds per square inch. If you open your mouth underwater, water flows in. When you open your mouth in a room, air flows in. Why? Atmospheric Pressure pushes air into your mouth until mouth pressure equals room pressure. Now inhale. Two sets of muscles enlarge your chest cavity. The *Intercostal Muscles* (think meat on spareribs) contract to lift your ribs up & out. That increases the chest **size**.

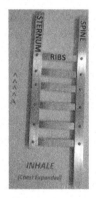 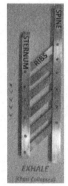 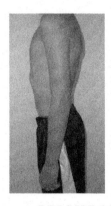 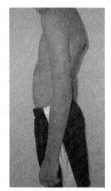

CHEST BREATHING   **BELLY BREATHING**

The *Diaphragm* is the dome-shaped muscle separating the chest and abdomen. When it contracts it flattens down toward the belly. This also expands the chest cavity. Standing, we mostly chest breathe. Lying down, we belly breathe. When sitting, we do a little of each.

INHALING - EXHALING

As the chest expands, air molecules inside bounce around in a bigger space. That means lower pressure. To equalize, atmospheric pressure pushes new air molecules into your mouth and down into your lungs. Congratulations, you just inhaled. The tough part of breathing is done.

Now relax, you'll exhale with no work at all. Intercostal and diaphragm muscles go limp and the chest collapses back to its smaller size. Same number of gas molecules bouncing around in a smaller space means higher pressure. That pressure equalizes out your nose and mouth. (Great design: Inhaling is fast work. Exhaling is slow relaxation, about twice as long as inhaling. That means you get to relax about 2/3's of your life.) Interesting, lifting the ribs to take in air is called *Chest Breathing*. Flattening the diaphragm is *Belly Breathing*. During sitting and standing, chest breathing is dominant. When lying down or sleeping, belly breathing does most of the work.

WHAT DO WE INHALE AND WHY? Here's another easy one. We breathe in the air all around us. On Earth, air is about 78% nitrogen and 21% oxygen.[1] (Forget the last 1%). For us, inhaled nitrogen is an *Inert Gas*. It doesn't chemically react. But, that 21% Oxygen, **that's** the key.

Experiment: Take a deep breath. Hold your breath while you answer this question. "What's **the** most essential nutrient for the human body?" Before you turn blue, the answer is **Oxygen**. How essential is it? Without oxygen, you're dead in 5-6 minutes. Why is it essential? Think about your car. Cars use spark plugs to burn fuel, **if** there's enough oxygen to support combustion. Your car won't run on the moon. There's not enough oxygen. Humans also require oxygen to burn our fuel (glucose).

WHAT DO WE EXHALE AND WHY? When we relax, we exhale. Exhaling empties 3 gases into the room. Nitrogen comes back out unchanged. We don't use all that 21% oxygen, so some of that also gets exhaled. But, the **big deal** for exhaling is carbon dioxide - CO_2 Just like your car, the result of burning fuel is ENERGY and CO_2.

$$\text{C-H-O} + O_2 = \text{ENERGY} + CO_2 + H_2O$$

**FUEL + OXYGEN = ENERGY + CARBON
DIOXIDE + WATER (vapor)**

Remember 'Global Warming' from 'TIPS' ? Sure hope you've cut back on all that exhaling...

One last point: Cars can't burn their fuel as completely as people do. So, car exhaust contains some carbon **mon**oxide, not just carbon **di**oxide.

———————

————

All that's normal. What happens when breathing goes wrong?

U.R.I.

Definition: URI means an **U**pper **R**espiratory **I**nfection from a virus. URI's used to be called colds. *Colds* was a funny name since they have nothing to do with cold weather, damp feet, or getting wet, despite what your grandmother told you. Colds were miserable, not dangerous, and lasted about 2 weeks. No treatment really worked. How common was the Common Cold? About 10 per year in kids and about 3 per year in adults![3] Seniors got the fewest (see below). None of that has changed. But...

Now, the formal diagnosis is **URI**. That acronym seems to give colds more importance somehow. Doctors really need to **do** something about URI's. Unfortunately, we have. We've done lots of things **wrong**. We now recommend or prescribe everything from vitamins to supplements to antibiotics. Those include Vitamin C, Vitamin D, Vitamin E, Echinacea, antibiotics like azithromycin (The Z Pack) and the entire 3 shelves of 'Cough and Cold' remedies at your local pharmacy. **All** of these have been tested in large clinical research trials. **None** has been found to prevent, lessen, or shorten the Common Cold.[4,5,6,7,8,]

You're still miserable for 12-14 days. You're still coughing for over 2 weeks.[9] Natural honey may help the cough.[10,11] Tylenol or NSAIDS may help aches and fever. Otherwise, don't make any serious plans for the next few weeks.

Germ Clue #1: Bacteria usually infect **one** place and need antibiotics. Examples: infected cut, strep throat, pneumonia, appendicitis, etc.

Germ Clue #2: Viruses make you sick all over and should **not** get antibiotics. Examples: colds, URI's, Flu, HIV, etc. Good news? Once you get over this cold virus, you'll never get it again. You're now immune to that one. Bad news? A couple hundred viruses cause URI's[12]. So, you're nose is clogged, throat's sore, voice is hoarse, head and body ache, and you're coughing all the time. My suggestions?

Treat aches and fever with Tylenol (generic is *Acetaminophen)* or Aleve (generic is *Naproxen)*

To protect others, wash your hands often and cough on your sleeve.

Lessen the cough with old fashioned honey[13,14]

Don't make serious plans for the next 2 weeks.

Finally, for doctors who rationalize using antibiotics for colds: "At least it prevents patients from developing Community Acquired Pneumonia". True, but very misleading. Case Western Reserve studied 814,283 patients. 65% of those got antibiotics for their URI's. Result? Taking an antibiotic **did** prevent pneumonia hospital admissions. How often? **One** prevented pneumonia for every **12,255** antibiotic prescriptions.

—————

————

INFLUENZA (The Flu)

Definition: a dangerous respiratory infection from a **preventable** virus. Influenza is 'The Cold from Hell'. Same Cold symptoms, but much worse: high fever, pounding headache, sore throat, aching muscles, and severe coughing. Sometimes there's even vomiting and diarrhea (remember, viruses infect your whole body). How bad is it? Influenza kills 35,000 – 40,000 Americans every year,[15] about the same as breast cancer. Let's start with Flu Shots: Up to 80% protection from one yearly shot[16] ; Costs about $25[17] ; Protects against both Influenza A and Influenza B[18] ; Side effects are usually minor. Needle Phobia? Now there's a nasal form[19]; "Egg Allergy?" Another new form is even safe for you[20]. And last, **No**, you cannot get Influenza from the Flu Shot[21]. Yet each year, 50-60% of us don't get a flu shot[22]. File under: Really Dumb. Why a new flu shot every year? Because Flu viruses are smart. "Hmmm…couldn't infect many people last season. Damn Flu shots. Better mutate this Spring so I can infect everybody next year." Remember "Vaccines" in Chapter 5? A vaccination is exposure to a **harmless** protein that looks like a germ.

For Influenza, the vaccine includes fakes of the prior 2 years' dominant flu strains plus the new strain from last Spring. The virus strains are either killed or made inactive, so they're harmless. But, your body can't tell these from the real virus. So, you make new Antibodies for each strain. This once a year Flu shot can give up to 80% protection against Influenza and its complications. Imagine if we had a once yearly vaccine that protected 80% of women from breast cancer.

QUESTION: "I never remember to get the shot. If I get the flu, can't I just take some pills?"

Sure! Once you're sick with Influenza, you can take Tamiflu pills (*oseltamivir* about $110)[23] or Relenza inhaler (*zanamivir* about $60)[24]. Results? Really work best if started in the first 48 hrs. That's when most people think, "It's just a cold." May prevent some flu complications. But, medicines only shorten your illness by about 1 ½ days![25]

"OK, but what about side effects? Can't you get that terrible *Guillain Barre* from a Flu shot?"

Yes…**but,** this rare nerve and muscle disease is 15 times more likely from Influenza (1 in 60,000) than from the Flu Shot (1 in 971,000)[26].

ASTHMA

Definition: Reversible shortness of breath from UNNECESSARY airway constriction and inflammation.

Asthma's kind of like Congress, a few really good ideas carried **way** too far. Suppose I'm trapped in a burning building. Flames, smoke, and superheated air all around me. I **don't** have asthma. My lungs have 3 defenses:

- Airway muscles constrict to reduce incoming heat and smoke.
- White blood cells rush to my lungs to begin clearing debris.
- Inflammation fluids make it easier to cough out that debris.

If I get out in time, constricted airways and inflammation just saved my life.

Now, I'm an asthma patient. This time it's not a house fire. It's just a smoky barroom or somebody's cat. Asthmatic brain says, "Emergency! Emergency! Constrict all airways. Send in the clean-up crew. Begin coughing." Symptoms are what you'd expect. "My chest is tight." "I get short of breath doing anything." "I'm always coughing and *wheezing*." Wheezing is a high pitched whistle at end of exhale. In your doctor's office, asthma testing is easy. The most common method is the ***FEV₁***.[27] FEV stands for **F**orced **E**xpiratory **V**olume. The little "₁" stands for 1 second. How much air can you can forcibly exhale in 1 second? If you don't exhale enough air, you get 2 puffs of an asthma inhaler. Wait 5 minutes. Doctor repeats your FEV_1. If the inhaler got your test back to normal, you have asthma.

Usually, other testing isn't necessary. Chest x-rays don't show constricted airways. Oxygen levels don't drop until you're critical. Allergy tests can have both false positive and false negative results.[28] Asthmatic lungs over-react to many things: cold, stress, exercise, infection, etc. Asthma is **not** just an allergy problem.

Asthma treatment should be easy:

Avoid triggers that bring on wheezing.

Use 2 puffs of a hand-held *Metered Dose Inhaler (MDI)* to inhale A*lbuterol* – a drug that relaxes airway muscles when an asthma attack starts;

Use a daily hand-held *Steroid* inhaler (reduces inflammation) to lessen chronic asthma attacks.

If it's that simple, why is asthma such a big deal? 3 reasons: Patients **like** their triggers - smoking is a great example. Patients **delay** using their albuterol inhaler, often from embarrassment. And, patients **don't** use their inhalers correctly.[29]

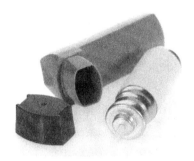

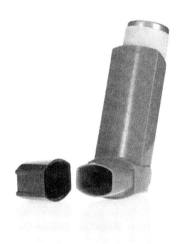

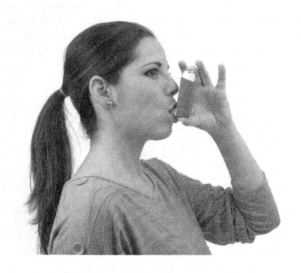

QUESTION: "What's the **right** way to use an inhaler?"

Assemble the inhaler, shake it up, remove cap.

Take a deep breath in and fully exhale.

Place inhaler in front of your open mouth.

Start a big inhale thru your mouth.

Put inhaler opening between your lips.

Mid-way through inhale, trigger the MDI.

Finish inhale.

Hold your breath as long as you can.

Wait 2-5 minutes and repeat the entire sequence.

Finally, ask your doctor about a **spacer** – there are many kinds. A spacer goes between your lips and the inhaler. It allows the medicine to aerosolize better before you inhale it, making it more effective.[30]

PNEUMONIA

Definition: a **dangerous** infection of the lungs' tiny air sacs – the *Alveoli.* Those air sacs are the **only** way oxygen enters the blood. Fill them with fluid or pus and no oxygen gets in. On chest x-ray, the area turns white. Both bacteria and viruses can cause pneumonia. Anatomy? The lungs have 5 lobes, 3 on the right and 2 on the left.

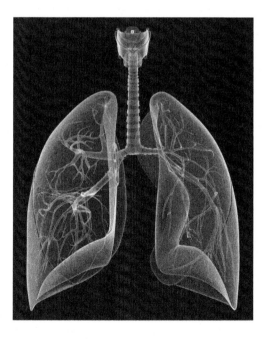

Lobar pneumonia means one infected lobe turns white on x-ray. *Double pneumonia* - 2 infected lobes. *Bilateral pneumonia* - at least one lobe on each side.

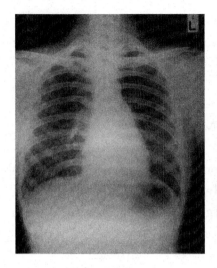 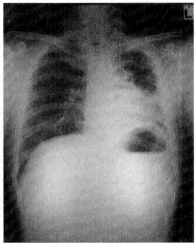

NORMAL **LEFT PNEUMONIA**

Symptoms? - These people are very sick. Fever, shaking chills, short of breath, painful coughing, even painful breathing.

How serious? - Very serious! 2- 3 million Americans develop pneumonia each year. About 45,000 of them will die[37].

Types? - I'll only cover *Community Acquired Pneumonia* here. Infections picked up in hospitals or nursing homes are worse – but beyond this book.

Causes? - Infants, children, adults, and seniors tend to get pneumonia from different germs.

Virus or Bacteria? - Virus infections should **not** get antibiotics. But, with pneumonia, there's no quick way to tell a virus from a bacteria. So, all pneumonias get antibiotics.

Treatment? - Very complicated. First, germs for each age group overlap. Second, many of our best antibiotics were 'wasted' on viral diagnoses like bronchitis and sinusitis[38]. This led to *Antibiotic Resistance* - smart bacteria just mutate to become resistant. Example? 10 years ago azithromycin was great for pneumonia. Now, at our local hospital, 48% of *Strep. Pneumoniae* (most common pneumonia bacteria) are resistant to it. [39]

Out Patient vs. In Patient? Patient seems very sick, **admit to hospital**. Patient has other health problems, **admit**. Patient's a long time smoker, **admit**. Unsure patient can comply with treatment, **admit**.

Why? Because pneumonia kills. Fever goes up. Pulse goes up. Respirations go up. Yet oxygen goes down until the brain drifts off to sleep, and death. For generations, Pneumonia's nickname was 'The Old Man's Friend' – a quiet, painless end of life. Sad, but still true.

———————

———

EMPHYSEMA and COPD (Chronic Obstructive Pulmonary Disease)

Definition: Irreversible inflammation and destruction of the lungs from smoking. (Yes, 1% of these patients inherit a bad gene. A few work in toxic factories, like cadmium. 3rd World women cook over indoor fires their whole lives, etc.) But, for everybody else, the cause is tobacco smoke. Names like Phillip Morris, Reynolds America, Lorillard, and the rest of the Tobacco Industry need to accept blame for our 3rd leading cause of death. (Emphysema and COPD are technically different, but the difference is too technical for this book.) Either way, the patient becomes ever more short of breath until he dies with these incurable diseases.

"Back to the Future"

- YEAR: 2050
- PLACE: 1ˢᵗ year medical school classroom
- LECTURE: "The History of Medicine"
- Professor: "50 years ago, tobacco was the #1 cause of heart attack, stroke, cancer, and emphysema. Those 4 diseases used up the majority of our healthcare budget. Lobbying by the Tobacco Industry kept it legal."
- Medical Student (giggling): "Wait, are you saying tobacco was **legal** in the United States?"
- Rest of students erupt in laughter at such a crazy thought.

Unfortunately, tobacco is legal, highly addictive[32], and very profitable.[33] To understand its lung effects, let's review some anatomy.

The Respiratory System

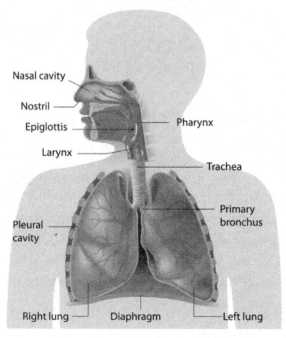

The upper airway includes the *Larynx* (voice box), the *Trachea* (windpipe), the *Right Main Bronchus,* and the *Left Main Bronchus.* These are the large breathing tubes to carry air down into the lungs. All these are made of tough cartilage and pretty durable.

Inside the lungs, cartilage is replaced by tubes with muscular walls. Finally, the smallest airways are just connective tissue ending in *Alveoli* – microscopic air sacs. During inhale, these muscular and connective tissue airways open slightly to allow air in. To exhale, they collapse, **in sequence**, to slowly squeeze the air back out. The upper airways also have fine hair cells (*Cilia)* that act like brooms to sweep dust and debris back out. How does smoking cause COPD? The 'Tobacco Villain' has 2 weapons. Over time, toxic smoke kills those hair cells. Ever notice how hard emphysema patients cough? Coughing is the only clearing method they have left. And smoking gradually destroys the elastic walls of the small airways. This doesn't happen all at once. And, it's **not** in sequence. One little airway collapses here, another wears out over there. Now try to exhale. Your chest collapses, increasing pressure inside. That pressure squashes some of those weakened pipes closed **before** the air behind the obstruction can be exhaled. That's the "Obstructive" of COPD. That trapped air causes back pressure. Each breath increases that pressure. Behind the obstruction, those tiny air sacs, already weak from tobacco's inflammation, begin to balloon out. Then they burst, one into another. These form *Blebs or Bullae,* useless groups of ruptured air sacs.

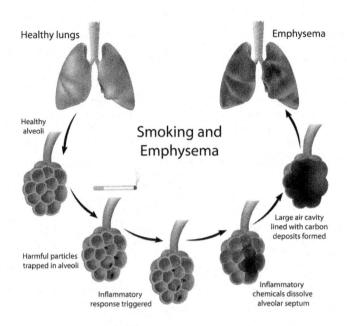

Healthy lungs — Emphysema

Healthy alveoli — Smoking and Emphysema

Harmful particles trapped in alveoli

Inflammatory response triggered

Inflammatory chemicals dissolve alveolar septum

Large air cavity lined with carbon deposits formed

Typical COPD Patient? Males more than females. Over age 50 (longer time to smoke). Whites more than Blacks or Hispanics. Poor more than their wealthy, better educated counterparts.[34] How much smoking does it take? A *pack year* means smoking 1 pack of cigarettes per day for 1 year. After 20 pack years, 15-20% of patients will develop COPD[35]. Since smokers often start in their teens, 20 pack years is common. In fact, the largest growth in smoking today is among teenagers[36]

Symptoms? The first symptom is cough. Does your smoker's cough bring up junk most days for 2 consecutive years? You just made your diagnosis. Trapped air that can't be exhaled increases the chest size. Now, you get no rest. You work to inhale and work even harder to exhale. The inflammation, airway weakening, and destruction of air sacs cause progressive shortness of breath. That continues until death.

Treatment? Remember, COPD, including Emphysema and Chronic Bronchitis, are incurable diseases. Some inhalers help relieve wheezing.

Other inhalers reduce inflammation. Portable oxygen tanks provide comfort to delay the inevitable.

Cure? Stopping smoking helps symptoms and delays progression. The only **cure** is a lung transplant.

TRAUMA: CRASHES, FALLS, AND BULLETS

You probably don't think of Trauma as a disease. Well, you should. If you're under 45, it's the disease most likely to kill you. It snuffs out over 34,000 American lives every year. We spend over $400 billion annually for Trauma's medical care and lost productivity[1]. But, Trauma is unique among human diseases – no warning, no immunizations, and no cure.

MVA stands for Motor Vehicle Accident – a car crash. Since that's our #1 cause of Trauma deaths, let's start there.

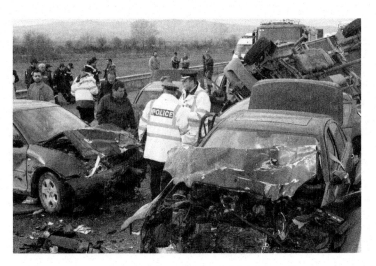

MOTOR VEHICLE ACCIDENTS

50 years ago, car crashes were the #1 Trauma fatality. Since then, the auto industry has made great strides in vehicle safety. We've gone from glass windshields to safety glass. From no seat belts to lap belts. From

lap belts to 3 point restraints. From no air bags to front air bags. And now, to front, side, and even some ceiling air bags. New tech devices keep us in our lane, warn of vehicles in our 'blind spot', and even brake to prevent an impending crash. The result? Car crashes are still our #1 Trauma deaths[2].

C'mon people, what are we missing here? Actually, we're missing 3 things.

Science: Heavy things moving fast have a lot of force. Simply put, a truck going 60 mph hits you harder than a compact car going 30 mph. It also takes more force to stop that truck, either with its brakes or by hitting you.

Marketing: Do we all really need pickup trucks to drive to the office? In 2013, we bought 50% more trucks than cars or SUV's. The 'Big 3' sellers are usually: Ford F-150 (pickup truck), Toyota Camry (car), and Honda's CRV (SUV).[3] Let's look at their specs. Toyota Camry weighs 1.62 tons.[4] Honda CRV weighs 1.71 tons.[5] Ford's F-150 weighs **2.34** tons.[6] At 60 mph, the lighter Car and SUV stop in about 120 feet. Pickup trucks are heavier and take a longer distance to stop, usually 1-3 more car lengths.[7] Question for pickup drivers: Why can't you guys remember that when you're driving behind me? (Remember, stopping distances compare vehicles, not different drivers' reaction times. At 60 mph, each second of reaction time equals 88 **more** feet of stopping distance.)

'Nut Behind the Wheel':

- 3 point seat belts reduce crash deaths by **50%**. 15% of us still won't wear them.
- 1/3 of all crash deaths are either alcohol or drug related.
- Use your cell phone while you drive?[8] You're **4 times** more likely to crash. Your teen tells you her better eyesight and faster

reflexes cancel that out. Wrong! Only 6% of U.S. drivers are 15-20 years old. Yet they account for 10% of MVA deaths and 13% of crash injuries.[9]

- Texting while driving? An average text message takes her eyes off the road for 4 seconds. At 60 mph, her car travels more than a football field in that time. How bad is that? In 2009, Eddie Alterman published a fascinating experiment in "Car and Driver" magazine. Conclusion: "texting while driving has a worse impact on safety than if you were driving while intoxicated."[10]
- One final word. **NO!** Hands free phones do not lower those risks.[11]

QUICK QUESTIONS:

Q: Most common Motor Vehicle Accident?

A: Being hit in the rear by the 'nut' behind you who doesn't know his stopping distance.

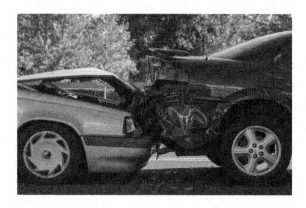

Q: Why do airbags save adults and kill kids?

A: At impact, an air bag must be fully inflated before you slam your face into it. To do that, they don't just open. Two chemicals inside

explode them open at nearly 200 mph, "the equivalent of a solid rocket booster"[12] . That opening force can easily kill small children in the front seat. Why?

Multiple reasons:

- Forward-facing child seats move the child closer to the deploying bag.
- In Rear-facing child seats, the opening bag crushes the back of the car seat into the back of the child's head.
- Direct seating in the front may be even worse. Short arms and legs can't reach out to brace before impact.
- Children are more likely to lean up and forward to see out.
- Shorter stature puts a child's head closer to the exploding bag than an adult's.
- Shoulder belts don't fit kids well. Slipping an arm out and over that part compromises the remaining lap belt. It also leaves **no** restraint for the torso, head, and neck.

SOLUTION? During a crash, the safest place in any vehicle is restrained in the middle of the back seat.

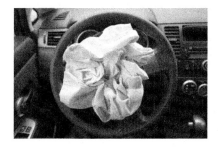
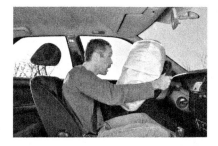

EXPLODING AIR BAG   **FULLY INFLATED AIR BAG**

JUST A THOUGHT: For all you folks who insist you have the **right** to refuse seat belts, motorcycle helmets, etc. OK, that's fine. Just please sign the **new** waiver on your Driver's License: "If I crash my car while not wearing my seat belt, or my motorcycle without my helmet on, I understand all medical care ends when my personal resources have been exhausted."

———————

————

FALLS (At ground level and from height)

Background: In 2010, 22,000 Americans died from falls. They're the leading cause of head injury in the elderly (over age 65) and the leading cause of hip fractures. 20% of patients with hip fractures die within one year. Probably 50% are dead within 2 years. Every year, about 30% of seniors suffer a fall. In 2010, that was 2.3 million falls with direct medical costs over $30 **billion**.[13] What height fall is deadly? An old formula said a fall from 3 times your own height killed 50%. Actually, falls have too many variables for simple numbers. Falling 2 stories and landing feet first in the water is very different from falling 10 feet head first onto concrete. The most common Trauma from falls are head injuries and fractures.

Head Injuries

Head injuries from falls are usually *Closed Head Injuries – CHI's*. CHI mean any head injury that does **not** penetrate the skull. Think of the skull as a China bowl filled with Jello. The 'Jello' is your brain. It's attached to the skull by fibrous tissue loaded with blood vessels.

CHI's come in 3 types:

#1. Brain is bruised and bleeding right under the point of injury on the scalp – like being hit by a baseball bat.

#2. Rapidly moving head is suddenly stopped by impact. Brain continues moving forward. Brain slams into skull – typical football injury.

#3. Sudden, severe skull **rotation**. Brain lags behind. Brain connections to skull are torn – like a boxer's left hook.

(SEE NEXT 3 PAGES FOR ILLUSTRATIONS OF EACH TYPE)

CLOSED HEAD INJURY #1

Direct Blow to Skull

SKULL

TINY BLOOD VESSELS

BRAIN

CRACKED SKULL

BRAIN

BLEEDING

BRUISED BRAIN

CLOSED HEAD INJURY #2

Sudden Stop (Fall or Car Crash)

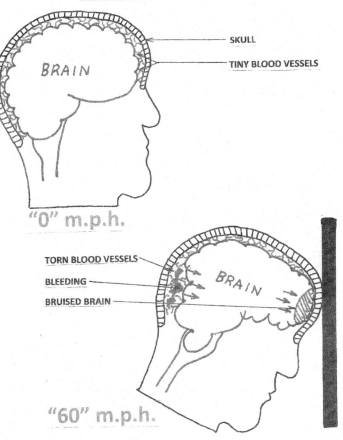

CLOSED HEAD INJURY #3

Sudden Skull Rotation ("Left Hook")

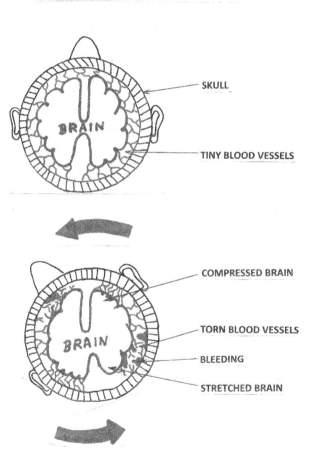

Common Fractures

- **Broken Wrist** – Probably the most common adult fracture. Falling onto an outstretched hand bends the wrist backward until it breaks **any** of the 10 bones at the wrist. Treatment: straighten the bones and cast for 6-8 weeks.

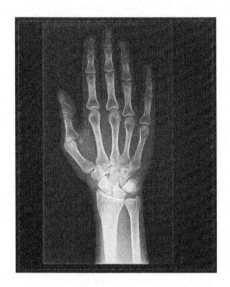 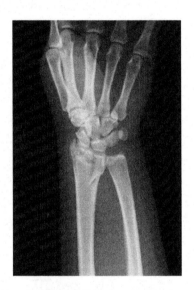

NORMAL WRIST   **BROKEN WRIST**

Spine Compression Fracture – falling onto the buttocks bends the spine forward until a vertebra gets squashed from above and below. Treatment: usually rest, but corrective surgery with hardware is becoming more common.

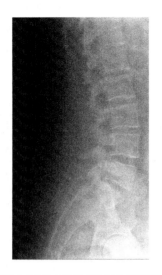 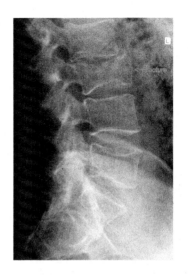

NORMAL LUMBAR SPINE   BROKEN LUMBAR SPINE

- **Broken Hip** – SHARP HIP ANGLE + OSTEOPOROSIS + FALL = **FRACTURE**. If the bone is really thin, the hip may even break spontaneously, without a fall. Treatment: surgery - ASAP. Period.

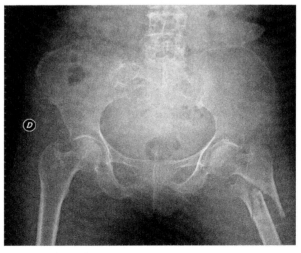

NORMAL HIP   BROKEN HIP

- **Broken Collar Bone** *(Clavicle)* – Probably the most common childhood fracture. Treatment: maybe just a sling for 4-6 weeks but some need surgery.

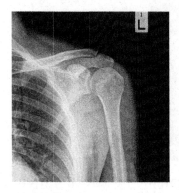
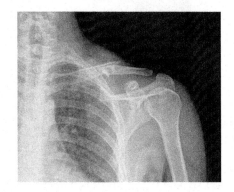

NORMAL COLLAR BONE   **BROKEN COLLAR BONE**

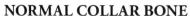

BULLETS

GSW is medical jargon for **G**un **S**hot **W**ounds. GSW's are America's #3 cause of deaths not from disease. (Motor Vehicle Accidents and Poisonings are #1 and #2.) In 2010, 31,513 Americans died from gunshot wounds. Of these deaths, about 19,000 were suicides, 11,000 were homicides, and 600 were accidental gunshot deaths[14].

Contrary to the anti-gun lobby, America is not returning to the days of the Wild West. Yes, we're #3 in the world for most deaths by guns. But, subtract Baltimore, Washington D.C., Chicago, and New Orleans. Then, America actually ranks 4th **from the bottom of the list.** Luckily, most people only see gun violence on TV. I call that 'Cinderella Violence'. Why?

Cinderella was a poor, unattractive young woman with no good life ahead of her. One quick visit from her Fairy God Mother. Suddenly she's a beautiful princess living happily ever after. Well, when **you** get shot on TV, **you're** Cinderella – complete with your own Fairy Godmother. **Why?**

TV's "Covert Affairs" had a great example of this. In a season finale, Annie Walker, the CIA heroine, is shot twice, mid-chest, with a 9mm handgun fired from about 6 ft. away. Next season, she wears low cut tops so you can see the two scars. Time out. Reality check. If poor Annie had she been shot **at** your local Shock Trauma Unit, it's highly unlikely she would have survived.

Ballistics is the scientific "study of the dynamics and flight characteristics of projectiles".[15] Bullets and shotgun pellets are high speed projectiles capable of going through human tissue. This is **not** good if you're one they are going through.

Let's look at 4 common bullets.

The Ammunition

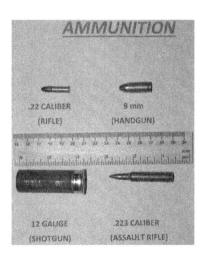

The Damage

Now let's look at what those bullets can do. The targets are one foot lengths of 2x4 lumber shot from a distance of 10 ft.

MEDICAL REMINDER: 2x4's are much tougher than your body.

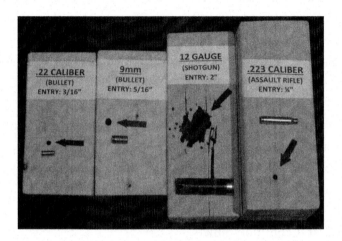

ENTRY ‹WOUNDS›

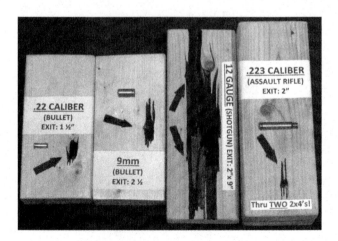

EXIT ‹WOUNDS›

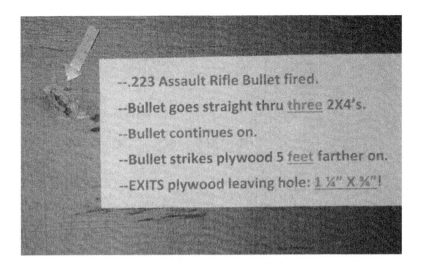

--.223 Assault Rifle Bullet fired.

--Bullet goes straight thru <u>three</u> 2X4's.

--Bullet continues on.

--Bullet strikes plywood 5 <u>feet</u> farther on.

--EXITS plywood leaving hole: <u>1 ¼" X ¾"</u>!

That's the science of bullets. How about a couple human questions?

Q: You're at home. An intruder with an assault rifle breaks in. Where should you hide?

A: Inside your car…in another town! Look at the photo above. That .223 assault bullet went thru three 2x4's, continued on 5 more feet, entered ½" plywood, then blew a 1 ¼" x ¾" hole out the back of the plywood!

Q: What's the safest place to get shot? On TV, good guys get shot all the time. ("Gunsmoke's" Sheriff Matt Dillon was shot over 100 times during the series.) So, where do they get shot?

A: Usually they 'only' get shot in the arm. Oops, slight medical problem…. Below, I've drawn a cross section of your arm, about mid biceps. Try to make a thru and thru bullet wound that won't wipe out that arm for good.

UPPER ARM ANATOMY

"He only got shot in the arm!"

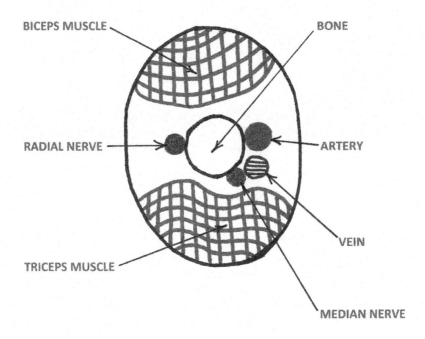

Last - a political hot potato. Jefferson inspired - and Madison wrote - our Bill of Rights. That includes our 2nd Amendment - "The right to bear arms". Back then, arms meant single shot rifles and pistols. Do you really think they meant today's assault rifles with high capacity magazines?

GLOSSARY

A1-C : Indirect measure of blood sugar over prior 3 months. (normal = less than 5.7%)

ABSTRACT: Summary of a medical journal article – usually available on-line.

ACETAMINOPHEN: Generic for Tylenol and less expensive.

ACETYLSALICYLIC ACID: Chemical name for aspirin.

ACUTE MYOCARDIAL INFARCTION: Heart Attack (see below).

AEROBIC INFECTION: Infection from bacteria that require oxygen to live.

ANAEROBIC INFECTION: Infection from bacteria that don't need oxygen.

ANEMIA: Too few Red Blood Cells.

ANNULUS FIBROSIS: Tough outer ring of a disc between vertebrae.

ANTIBODY: Immune system protein designed to engulf a specific antigen (see below).

ANTICOAGULANTS: medicines that slow down blood clotting (also called blood thinners).

ANTIGEN: Foreign protein causing an immune response in the body.

ARTERIOSCLEROSIS: Hardening (narrowing) of the arteries by fatty deposits.

ARTHRITIS: Inflammation of a joint.

ASTHMA: Disease that constricts and inflames breathing pipes in the lungs.

ATRIUM: The 2 upper chambers of the heart – Right Atrium and Left Atrium

ATMOSPHERIC PRESSURE: Weight of the Earth's atmosphere.

ATRIAL FIBRILLATION: Abnormal heart rhythm when the upper chambers wiggle instead of pump.

AUTO-IMMUNE DISORDER : Body develops immunity against normal body tissue.

BETA BLOCKERS: Medicines used to slow fast heart rhythms and lower high blood pressure.

BETA CELLS : Pancreas cells that produce insulin.

BMI (Body Mass Index): Estimate of body fat. Normal=19-25, Overweight=25-30, Obese=30+.

BRONCHUS: Cartilage breathing tubes from the windpipe into the lungs.

BRUIT: Sound of turbulent blood passing thru a narrowed artery.

BURSA: Collapsed water balloon to pad bony angles (knee, elbow, hip, etc.).

BURSITIS: Inflamed bursa.

CABG: Coronary Artery Bypass Graft (see below).

CAPILLARIES: Tiny blood vessels between the end of an artery and the beginning of a vein.

CARDIAC ARREST: Complete heart stoppage with no blood being pumped.

CARDIAC CATHETERIZATION: Thin tube slid into a heart blood vessel for x-ray or procedure.

CARDIAC ENZYMES: Specific heart proteins that may leak into the blood after a heart attack.

CARDIO-PULMONARY ARREST: Complete stoppage of breathing and heartbeat.

CARDIO-PULMONARY RESUSCITATION: Various temporary techniques to circulate blood and artificially breathe for a patient after a Cardiac-Pulmonary Arrest. CPR for short.

CAROTID ARTERIES : 2 arteries in the front of the neck that are the brain's major blood supply.

CARTILAGE: Shiny, slippery tissue covering bone ends.

CDC: Centers for Disease Control & Prevention (adding cdc to web search improves results).

CHF: Congestive heart Failure (see below).

CEREBROVASCULAR ACCIDENT (CVA) : A stroke.

CERVICAL SPINE: Top 7 vertebrae - neck portion of the spine.

CHOLESTEROL: Fatty chemical made in the liver, essential for all body cells, and previously believed to be the cause of heart attacks and strokes.

CHRONIC OBSTRUCTIVE PULMONARY DISEASE: Lung elastic tissue essential for *exhaling* is destroyed by smoking.

CLAVICLE: Collar bone.

CORONARY ARTERY BYPASS GRAFT: Small section of arm or leg vein used to surgically bypass a blockage in a heart artery.

C.O.P.D.: Chronic Obstructive Pulmonary Disease (see above).

COCCYX: Tailbone.

CONGESTIVE HEART FAILURE: Heart's too weak to pump out the blood coming in to it.

CORONARY ARTERIES: Two small arteries that supply the heart.

CONTRAINDICATIONS: medical conditions or reasons when a drug cannot be used.

CONTUSION: Bruise.

COUMADIN: Oldest and most widely used blood thinner – also called Warfarin.

CVA: Abbreviation for Cerebro-Vascular Accident – a Stroke.

DELUSION: Unreal thought.

DEPRESSION: Depleted brain chemicals make patients feel hopeless, helpless, and worthless.

DIABETES MELLITUS: Sugar Diabetes (mellitus is honey in Latin) – too high blood sugar from too little insulin for body size.

DIAPHRAGM: Dome-shaped respiratory muscle between the lower chest and upper belly.

DIASTOLIC BLOOD PRESSURE: Lower of the 2 numbers in a blood pressure reading.

DISLOCATION: Bone ends come apart at a joint.

DIURETICS: Medicines that increase urine output to help blood pressure, heart failure, edema (swelling), glaucoma, etc.

ECHOCARDIOGRAM: A sonogram of the heart to check the valves and blood flow.

EJECTION FRACTION: % of blood in heart that it pumps out with each beat.

EKG: (see *Electrocardiogram* below).

ELECTROCARDIOGRAM: Test showing heart electricity from 12 different views.

EMBOLISM: Blood clot breaking free and traveling elsewhere.

EMPHYSEMA: Chronic lung inflammation and destruction from smoking.

EXTERNAL HEMORRHOID: Large intestine varicose vein just outside the anus.

F.E.V.$_1$: Amount you can forcibly exhale in 1 second.

FEMORAL ARTERY: Large right and left groin arteries supplying each leg.

FEMUR: The thigh bone.

FRACTURE: Broken bone.

FLU : Influenza.

FRUCTOSE: A simple sugar found in honey and many fruits.

GENERIC : Medication that's identical to a brand name product but less expensive.

GINGIVAL INFECTION: Gum infection, often from anaerobic germs (see above).

GINGIVITIS: Inflammation or infection of the gums.

GLUCOMETER: Small computer device to measure blood sugar.

GLUCOSE: A simple sugar and the body's primary fuel.

GLYCOGEN: 30,000 glucose molecules linked together for storage.

GLYCOLATED HEMOGLOBIN A1-C: See A1-C above.

HALLUCINATION: Unreal sensation like seeing or hearing that don't exist.

HEART ATTACK: Piece of heart muscle dies when its artery clots off.

HEMATOMA: Blood blister.

HEMAGLOBIN : Iron containing protein that fills Red Blood Cells and transports oxygen.

HEMAGLOBIN A1-C: See A1-C above.

HEMORRHOID: Varicose (distended) vein around the anus.

HERNIATED DISC: Soft center of vertebral disc squirts out from pressure.

HUMERUS: Upper arm bone.

HYPERTENSION: High blood pressure, usually from constricted body arteries.

INFLAMMATION : red, hot, painful, tender swelling designed for healing.

INFLUENZA : Serious respiratory virus – 80% prevented by the "Flu Shot".

INSULIN RESISTANCE : A theory of Type 2 Diabetes - body cells need more insulin to react normally.

INTERCOSTAL MUSCLES: Respiratory muscles between the ribs to lift the chest.

INTERNAL DEFIBRILLATOR: Surgically implanted electric device wired to the heart to shock it if the deadly Ventricular Fibrillation rhythm occurs.

INTERNAL HEMORRHOID: large intestine varicose vein just inside the anus.

- ITIS : Suffix meaning inflamed.

LARYNX: Voice box.

LEUKEMIA: Disabled, fast growing, cancerous white blood cells take over bone marrow.

LIGAMENTS: Tough soft tissue bands holding bones together at joints.

LUMBAR SPINE: 5 large vertebrae of the concave low back.

MAYO: Short for Mayo Clinic (adding mayo to web searches improves results).

METFORMIN: Type 2 Diabetes pill that lowers blood sugar by a) less sugar absorption by intestine, and b) stops liver from storing sugar as glycogen.

MITRAL VALVE STENOSIS: A narrowed heart valve slowing blood flow and sometimes producing clots.

MUSCULOSKELETAL SYSTEM: Body framework of bones, muscles, tendons, ligaments, cartilage, and joints.

MYOCARDIAL INFARCTION: Heart Attack.

N: The number of people in a study.

NAPROXEN: Generic for Aleve. Top orthopedists' NSAID choice and least cardiovascular risk.

NIH: Short for National Institutes of Health (adding nih to a web search improves results).

NSAID: Non-Steroid Anti-inflammation Drug.

NUCLEUS PULPOSUS: Jello-like filling of a vertebral disc that can herniate.

ORTHOPEDICS: Medical specialty diagnosing and treating injuries and illnesses of the musculoskeletal system.

ORTHOPEDIST: Doctor who specializes in Orthopedics (above).

PATELLA: Kneecap.

PLASMA: The yellowish liquid part of blood.

PLATELET: Tiny blood cell containing clotting chemicals.

PNEUMONIA: Lung infection when tiny air sacs fill with pus and germs.

PRE-DIABETES: Fasting blood sugar above normal 100 but below diabetic 125.

PRE-PATELLAR BURSA: Collapsed water balloon padding front of knee.

PULSE OX: % of Red Blood Cells carrying oxygen.

PULSE OXIMETER: Small digital device clipped to finger to measure pulse ox (see above).

PURPURA: Rash resembling large areas of bruising under the skin but without injury.

RBC: Abbreviation for Red Blood Cell.

RED BLOOD CELL: Round blood cell that transports oxygen.

RHEUMATIC FEVER: Rare, but dangerous complication of untreated strep infection.

RISK FACTORS: Life style or life events making a disease more likely (not necessarily a cause).

SACRUM/SACRAL SPINE: 5 fused lower spine bones between lumbar spine and tailbone.

SCAPULA: Shoulder blade.

SEPTIC ARTHRITIS: Very serious joint infection.

SHOCK: Blood pressure too low to supply oxygen and nutrients to tissues.

SLIPPED DISC: Soft center of vertebral disc squirts out from pressure.

SOFT TISSUE: All body tissues except bone (all soft tissue is gray on plain x-rays).

STATIN DRUGS: Cholesterol lowering drugs like Lipitor, Crestor, pravastatin, etc.

STENT: Compressed metal coil opened inside a blood vessel to keep it open.

SPRAIN: Stretching or tearing of ligaments holding bones together at joints.

STRAIN: Stretching or tearing of tendons holding muscles to bones.

STROKE: Piece of brain dies when its artery clots or bleeds.

SUCROSE: Table sugar —a complex sugar made of 50% glucose and 50% fructose.

SYSTOLIC BLOOD PRESSURE: Higher of the 2 numbers in a blood pressure reading.

TPA: (see Tissue Plasminogen Activator - below)

TENDONS: Soft tissue bands connecting muscles to bones.

TIBIA: Shin bone.

THORACIC SPINE: 12 back vertebrae between the neck and the low back.

TIA: Short for **T**ranscient **I**schemic **A**ttack, a temporary Stroke.

TISSUE PLASMINOGEN ACTIVATOR (TPA) : A medication given into a vein that dissolves blood clots.

TRACHEA: Windpipe.

TRANSCIENT ISCHEMIC ATTACK: Temporary stroke completely resolving in less than 24 hours.

TYPE 1 DIABETES: High blood sugar from a pancreas unable to produce insulin.

TYPE 2 DIABETES: High blood sugar when a pancreas can't make enough insulin for body size.

UPPER RESPIRATORY INFECTION: virus cold.

U.R.I.: Upper Respiratory Infection (see above).

V. FIB.: Short for the deadly heart rhythm, Ventricular Fibrillation (see below).

VENTRICLE: The 2 lower chambers of the heart – Right Ventricle and Left Ventricle.

VENTRICULAR FIBRILLATION: Deadly change in heart rhythm causing the Ventricles (2 lower heart chambers) to stop pumping and just wiggle.

WARFARIN: Oldest and most widely used anticoagulant – also called Coumadin.

WBC: Abbreviation for White Blood Cell (see below)

WHITE BLOOD CELL: Various kinds of blood cells involved with immunity and infection.

REFERENCES

(Whenever <u>The Merck Manual</u> is cited, it refers to <u>The MERCK Manual of Diagnosis and Therapy</u>, 19th Edition, Robert S. Porter, M.D.-editor, 2011)

TIPS

1. "Comparison of Weight Loss Diets with Different Composition of Fats, Proteins, and Carbohydrates", Sacks, Frank M., et. al., "New England Journal of Medicine", 360(9):859-873, 2/26/09.
2. "Wall Street Journal", 11/23/12.
3. "Pet Ownership Statistics", www.avma.org, 2012.
4. "Animal Bites", www.whoint/mediacentre/fact, 2/2013.
5. "Human Rabies", www.cdc.gov.
6. "Statement on Travellers and Rabies Vaccine", Canada Communicable Disease Report, Volume 28.ACS-4, 3/1/02.
7. Dental Professional Customer Service: Sonicare – 800-676-7664 and Waterpik – 800-525-2020.
8. "Comparison of Gingivitis Reduction and Plaque Removal by Sonicare Diamond Clean and a Manual Toothbrush", Delaurenti, M., et. al., "Journal of Dental Research", 91(special issue B):522, 2012.
9. "Cotton-tip Applicators as a Leading Cause of Otitis Externa", Nussinovitch, M., et. al., "International Journal of Otolaryngology", 68(4), 433-5, 4/2004.

10. "Analysis of the Literature: The Use of Mobile Phones While Driving", Brace, C.L., et. al. Monash University Accident Research Center, 4/17/07.

11. "Is a Hands-Free Phone Safer than a Handheld Phone", Ishigami & Klein, "Journal of Safety Research", 40: 157-164, 2009.

12. www.nhtsa.gov/driving, (Distracted Driving).

13. www.distraction.gov/content/get-the-facts

14. water.usgs.gov/edu/propertyyou

15. "Volume Depletion", The Merck Manual, 19th Edition, page 822.

16. newsok.com, 12/12/93.

17. "Ice Age", Wikipedia.

18. "Earth's Atmosphere", Wikipedia.

19. www.answers.com

20. Julius Caesar, Shakespeare, Wm., Act I, Scene 2, Lines 140-141.

21. The Merck Manual, pages 750-753.

22. American Melanoma Foundation, www.melanomafoundation.org

DIABETES

1. "2011 National Diabetes Fact Sheet"; Centers for Disease Control; Atlanta, Georgia. (number of American diabetics).

2. Same as #1. (number of American pre-diabetics).

3. www.healthyfellow.com

4. "Lack of Evidence of High Fructose Corn Syrup as the Cause of the Obesity Epidemic"; Klurfeld, D.L., et al.; "International Journal of Obesity"; 37(6): 771-773; 6/13.

5. "Evidence Based Review of the Effect of Normal Dietary Consumption (95th %) of Fructose on Hyperlipidemia and Obesity in Healthy, Normal Weight Individuals"; Dolan, Laurie

C., et al.; "Critical Reviews in Food Science and Nutrition"; Volume 50, Issue 1, 2009

6. "A Critical Review of the Evidence Relating High Fructose Corn Syrup and Weight Gain"; Forshee, R.A., et al.; "Critical Reviews in Food Science and Nutrition"; Volume 47, Issue 6, 2007.

7. "Deaths Among People with Diabetes, United States"; National Diabetes Information Clearing House, (a service of) The National Institutes of Health.

8. "Breast Cancer Statistics"; CDC home page; Centers for Disease Control and Prevention, Atlanta, Georgia

9. "The Cost of Diabetes – Results"; American Diabetic Association; www.diabetes.org .

10. National Diabetes Information Clearing House; National Institutes of Health; sugar levels chart.

11. "Cost of Self-Monitoring of Blood Glucose in the United States Among Patients on an Insulin Regimen for Diabetes"; Yeaw, J., et al.; "Journal of Managed Care Pharmacy"; 18 (1), 21-32; Jan/Feb 2012.

12. "How is the A1-C Used to Diagnose Type 2 Diabetes and Pre-Diabetes?"; National Diabetes Information Clearing House, (a service of the National Institutes Of Health).

13. "Comparison of Weight Loss Diets with Different Composition of Fat, Protein, and Carbohydrates"; Sacks, F.M., et al.; "New England Journal of Medicine"; 360(9): 859-873; 2/26/09.

14. "Treatments and Drugs"; Diseases and Conditions – Type 2 Diabetes; www.mayoclinic.org.

15. Wikipedia.com

TRANSLATING MEDICALESE

1. The Merck Manual 19th Edition; Porter, R.S. (Editor-in-Chief), p. 2861; 2011.
2. The Merck Manual 19th Edition; Porter, R.S. (Editor-in-Chief), p. 2861; 2011.
3. "The Sensitivity and Specificity of Rapid Antigen Testing in Streptococcal Upper Respiratory Infections"; Gurol, y.; et.al.; "International Journal of Pediatric Otorhinolaryngology"; 74(6): 591-593; 6/10.
4. CVS Minute Clinics website 11/14.
5. "Performance of a Rapid Strep Test and Throat Culture in Community Pediatric Offices – Implications for Management of Pharyngitis"; Tanz, R.R., et. al.; "Pediatrics", 123(2): 437-444; 2/09.
6. www.mdcalc.com/modified-centor-score-for-strep-pharyngitis
7. "Clinical Score and Rapid Antigen Detection Test to Guide Antibiotic Use for Sore Throats"; Little, P., et. al.; "British Medical Journal", 347: f5806; 10/10/13.
8. "Streptococcal Pharyngitis in Children – a Meta-analysis of Clinical Decision Rules and Their Clinical Variables"; Marechol, F.L., et. al.; "British Medical Journal", 3: e00, 1482; 3/9/13.
9. "Biochemical Testing of Thyroid Function"; Klee, G.G.; "Endocrinology and Metabolic Clinics of North America"; 26(4):765-775; 12/1997.
10. www.cdc.gov
11. www.cdc.gov
12. www.mayoclinic.org
13. "Short Term Outcomes of Prostate Biopsy in Men Tested for Cancer by Prostate Specific Antigen: Prospective Evaluation within Protect Study"; Rosario, D.J., et. al.; "British Medical Journal", 344:d7894; 1/9/12.
14. www.cdc.gov "Cancer Statistics by Type"

15. "Constipation, Laxative Use, and Risk of Colorectal Cancer: The Miyagi Cohort Study"; Watanabe, T., et. al.; "European Journal of Cancer"; 40(14), 2109-2115; 9/04.

16. "Constipation, Laxative Use, and Colon Cancer in a North Carolina Population"; Roberts, M.C., et. al.; "American Journal of Gastroenterology"; 98(4): 857-864; 4/03.

17. "Patients with Functional Constipation Do Not Have increased Prevalence of Colorectal Cancer Precursors"; Chan, Annie, et.al.; "GUT – International Journal of Gastroenterology and Hepatology"; 56(3): 451-452; 3/07.

ORTHOPEDICS

1. Methylprednisolone Injection for Carpal Tunnel Syndrome", Atoshi, I, et.al., "Annals of internal Medicine", 159(5): 309, 9/3/13

MEDICATIONS

1. "Facts about Generic Drugs", fda.gov, 9/12.
2. "Brand Names vs. Generic Drugs – Is One Better than the Other?"." newsnetwork.mayoclinic.org, 2/12.
3. Approximate cost for these OTC (Over the Counter) drugs at a national department store chain.
4. Micromedex^R Solutions, courtesy of my local hospital.
5. "Journal of Clinical Psycho-Pharmacology" 10/11.
6. "Content Analysis of false and Misleading Claims in television Advertising for Prescription and Nonprescription Drugs", Faeber, A.E., et. al., "Journal of General internal Medicine", 29(1): 110, 1/14.

7. "Dabigatran vs. Warfarin in Patients with Atrial Fibrillation", Connolly, S.J., et.al., "New England Journal of Medicine", 361: 1139-1151, 9/09.
8. Wikipedia
9. "Pharmacy Research and Development: What Do We Get for All That Money?", "British Medical Journal", 2012; 345: e 4348.
10. The Huffington Post, Alexander Eichler, 8/9/12.
11. "The Cost of Pushing Pills: a New Estimate of Pharmaceutical Promotion Expenditures in the U.S.", Gagnon, Marc-Andre, Lexchin, Joel, "PLOS Medicine", 1/3/08.
12. www.goodrx.com

LUNGS

1. Wikipedia, www.wikipedia.org
2. "We just gotta do sumthin' about carbon dioxide"; Bedard, Patrick; "Car & Driver"; 11/2002; p. 21.
3. a. "Upper Respiratory Tract Infections"; Cleveland Clinic Center for Continuing Education; www.clevelandclinicmeded.com (and) b. "Health Guide"; "New York Times"; 5/14/14; www.nytimes.com
4. www.mayoclinic.org
5. "Effect of Vitamin D3 Supplementation on Upper Respiratory Tract Infections in Healthy Adults – The Vidaris Randomized Controlled Trial"; Murdoch, D.R.; "JAMA"; 308(13):1333, 10/3/12.
6. "What the Science Says About Natural Products for the Flu and Colds"; Josephine P. Briggs, M.D. (Director, National Center of Complementary and Alternative Medicine); www.nccam.nih.gov ; 3/12/12 "Common Cold"; National Institute of Allergy and Infectious Disease; www.niaid.nih.gov

7. "Common Cold"; National Institute of Allergy and Infectious Disease; www.niaid.nih.gov

8. Cold/ Flu/ and Cough Health Center; www.webmd.com .

9. "How Long Does a Cough Last? Comparing Patients' Expectations with Data from a Systematic Review of the Literature"; Ebell, M.H.; et.al.; "Ann. Fam. Med."; 11(1):5, 1-2/13.

10. "Honey Plus Coffee Versus Systemic Steroid in Treatment of Persistent Post-Infectious Cough – a Randomized Controlled Trial"; Raeessi, M.A., et. al.; "Primary Care Respiratory Journal"; 22(3):325, 9/13.

11. "Therapeutic Options for Acute Cough Due to Upper Respiratory Infections in Children"; Paul, I.M.; "Lung"; 190(1):41, 2/12.

10. "Common Cold"; National Institute of Allergy and Infectious Disease; www.niaid.nih.gov

12. "Common Cold and Runny Nose", Centers for Disease Control, www.cdc.gov.

13. "A Comparison of the Effect of Honey, Dextromethorphan, and Diphenhydramine on Nightly Cough and Sleep Quality in Children and Their Parents"; Shadkam, M.N., et. al.; 7/10.

14. See References #5 and #6 above.

15. "Mandating Influenza Vaccination for Healthcare Workers"; Sullivan, S.J., et.al.; "Expert Rev. Vaccines"; 8(11): 11/09.

16 & 17. "Influenza Vaccine for 2013-2014"; "The Medical Letter", pp. 73-75; 9/16/13.

18. www.cdc.gov/flu

19. www.cdc.gov/flu/about/qa/nasalspray

20. www.flublok.com

21. "Misconceptions About Seasonal Flu and Flu Vaccines"; Centers for Disease Control; www.cdc.gov

22. "Flu Outbreak – Why are so many Americans Not Getting Vaccinated?"; Gush, Loren, Fox News; www.foxnews.com

23 & 24. "Antiviral Drugs for Influenza 2013-2014"; "The Medical Letter", pp.6-8, 1/20/14.

25. "Treatment Efficacy and Effectiveness Studies"; Centers for Disease Control, www.cdc.gov

26. "Risk of Guillain Barre' Syndrome After Seasonal Influenza Vaccine and Influenza Healthcare Encounters – a Self-Controlled Study"; Kwong, J.C., et.al.; "Lancet", 13(9):769, 5/13.

27. medical-dictionary.thefreedictionary.com

28. "Tests & Procedures – Results: Allergy Skin Tests"; The Mayo Clinic; www.mayoclinic.org

29. "Inhaler Misuse Remains Common in Real Life and is Associated with Reduced Disease Control"; Melani, A.S., et.al.; "Respiratory Medicine", 105(6):930, 6/11.

30. "How to Use an Inhaler with Spacer"; Med Line Plus, National Institutes of Health, www.nlm.nih.gov

31. The Merck Manual of Diagnosis and Therapy, 19th Edition, pp. 1889 & 1901.

32. "A Word About Success Rates for Quitting Smoking"; American Cancer Society; 2/6/14, www.cancer.org

33. "Global Profits for Tobacco Trade Total $35 Billion as Smoking Deaths Top 6 Million"; Simon Bowers; "The Guardian", 3/21/12; www.theguardian.com .

34. The Merck Manual of Diagnosis and Therapy, 19th Edition, p. 1891.

35. "COPD-The Silent Killer, Another Four Letter Word for Smoking"; Maloof, R.; "MSN Healthy Living"; healthyliving.msm.com .

36. "Preventing Tobacco Use Among Youth and Young Adults"; Sebelius, K. - Surgeon General Report, Dept. Health & Human Services; www.cdc.gov/tobacco ;2012.

37. The Merck Manual of Diagnosis and Therapy, 19th Edition, p. 1923.

38. "Principles of Appropriate Antibiotic Use for Treatment of Uncomplicated Acute Bronchitis"; Gonzales, R.; et. al.; "Ann. Int. Med.", 134(6), 521-9; 3/20/01. (See also NIH and Mayo Clinic websites listed above.)

39. "All Gram Positive Isolates, 2013 F.M.H. Antibiogram"; A. Belani, M.D.; 4/14.

TRAUMA

1. www.nationaltraumainstitute.org
2. www.cdc.gov/motorvehiclesafety
3. www.edmunds.com/car-reviews/top/10-10best-selling
4. www.toyota.com/camry/features
5. www.automobiles.honda.com/cr-v/specifications
6. www.ford.com/trucks/F150/specifications/capacities
7. www.google.com/search?q=truck+stopping+distance+vs+car&sa
8. "A Comparison of the Cell Phone Driver and the Drunk Driver", "Human Factors", 48(2), 381-91, Summer, 2006.
9. "Distracted Driving Raises Crash Risk", www.gov/researchmatters, 1/2014.
10. "Texting While Driving, How Dangerous Is It?", Eddie Alterman, "Car and Driver", 6/2009
11. www.nhtsa.gov/driving+safety/distracted
12. auto.howstuffworks.com/car
13. www.cdc.gov/homeandrecreationsafety/falls
14. www.pewresearch.org/fact-tank «Suicide Accounts for Most Gun Deaths"
15. Webster's II Dictionary, 3rd Edition, 7/05